Second Edition

WORKING WITH THE AGED

PRACTICAL APPROACHES IN THE INSTITUTION AND COMMUNITY

PART I

An Overview

Second Edition

WORKING WITH THE AGED

PRACTICAL APPROACHES IN THE INSTITUTION AND COMMUNITY

Second Edition

WORKING WITH THE AGED

PRACTICAL APPROACHES IN THE INSTITUTION AND COMMUNITY

Marcella Bakur Weiner, Ed.D.
Adjunct Professor
Fordham University Graduate School of Social Service
New York, New York

Former Senior Research Scientist
Gerontology/Sociology Division
New York State Department of Mental Hygiene

Albert J. Brok, Ph.D.
Faculty Supervisor
Postgraduate Center for Mental Health
New York, New York

Associate Clinical Professor
Adelphi University Postdoctoral Program in Group Psychotherapy
Garden City, New York

Alvin M. Snadowsky, Ph.D.
Professor of Psychology
Brooklyn College of the City University of New York
Brooklyn, New York

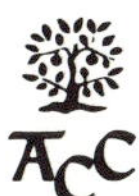

APPLETON-CENTURY-CROFTS / Norwalk, Connecticut

0-8385-9833-1

Notice: The author(s) and publisher of this volume have taken care that the information and recommendations contained herein are accurate and compatible with the standards generally accepted at the time of publication.

87 88 89 90 / 10 9 8 7 6 5 4 3 2 1

Prentice-Hall of Australia, Pty. Ltd., Sydney
Prentice-Hall Canada, Inc.
Prentice-Hall Hispanoamericana, S.A., Mexico
Prentice-Hall of India Private Limited, New Delhi
Prentice-Hall International (UK) Limited, London
Prentice-Hall of Japan, Inc., Tokyo
Prentice-Hall of Southeast Asia (Pte.) Ltd., Singapore
Whitehall Books Ltd., Wellington, New Zealand
Editora Prentice-Hall do Brasil Ltda., Rio de Janeiro

Library of Congress Cataloging-in-Publication Data

Weiner, Marcella Bakur, 1925–
Working with the aged.
Includes bibliographies and index.
I. Brok, Albert J. II. Snadowsky, Alvin M.,
1938– . III. Title. [DNLM: 1. Aged. 2. Aging.
3. Geriatrics—methods. 4. Rehabilitation—in old age.
WT 100 W423w]
RC954.W39 1987 610.73′65 86-14650
ISBN 0-8385-9833-1

Design: M. Chandler Martylewski
Cover: Kathleen Peters
Cover Photograph: Kathleen Peters

PRINTED IN THE UNITED STATES OF AMERICA

To my parents, Anna and Louis Shapiro, who taught me that aging could be upbeat.

Marcella Bakur Weiner

To the memory of my father, Benjamin Brok.

Albert J. Brok

To the memory of my parents, Florence and Jack Snadowsky.

Alvin M. Snadowsky

Contents

Preface

In offering this revised edition of *Working with the Aged*, we are hoping to acquaint new readers with the latest approaches for working with older people in institutional and community settings. To our readers already familiar with this material, we are providing the latest information on research in aging, along with new material on families as team members and on psychotherapy with older adults.

Despite the familiarity of some chapter headings, we feel that, in many ways, this is a new book geared to the worker wishing to understand both the theoretical aspects of aging and their practical application. We know now that many of the techniques described in the earlier version of this book work well and are still being used by those working with older persons. For those new to the field, we feel that our step-by-step guides will be helpful, providing the structure that newcomers need. It is our hope that those trying these techniques will eventually modify and improve upon them, as we ourselves have.

While the field of aging has exploded since our earlier edition, there are still few books that address issues relevant to both community- and institutional-living elderly. Though each population is distinct, there are similarities, as revealed in our chapters on physiological and psychological aging. Of increasing import are the family and the community-at-large, also addressed in this work.

This book has served a major need in the past, when the field of gerontology was relatively new. With this field now in its adulthood, this new edition can continue its role as a major text for multidisciplined persons working, or planning to work, with the elderly.

Acknowledgments

We are indebted to Dr. Miriam Aronson for her sensitive reading of the manuscript and for her helpful suggestions. Students Denise Lowe Brody, M.S.W.; Ann Marie Cornell, M.S.W.; and Sallie Lapa, M.S.W.; gave their time and efforts conscientiously, and we thank them. Susan Friedman, our typist, was always there with her gracious availability and skill. Our Editor, David Gordon, always took the time to confer with us and was supportive throughout. Production Editor Janice E. Yaeger treated our manuscript with the care that we felt it deserved. Finally, to all of the elderly with whom we worked, and whose needs prompted this book, we extend our heartfelt appreciation.

1

Why Work with the Aged?

THE MYTHOLOGY OF AGING

Ambivalences and contradictions are deeply imbedded in our attitudes toward aging. These attitudes are reflected in older people we know, those who are part of our private lives and feelings, and also in public attitudes toward those elderly "out there" or unknown to us. On the one hand, we see older people in general as demanding, debilitated, disagreeable, and a burden to their families. In contrast, we consider our own older relatives worthy of our affection and care.[1]

Where did these attitudes come from? Research shows that they are formed early in life. Children as young as three or four accept some of our common myths about aging. Shown a set of drawings of men of different ages, including older men, children aged three and four identified the oldest man as "wrinkled," "having no hair and teeth," and "ugly."[2] Yet, in another study, when children five and eight were shown photographs of people at different stages of life, ranging from childhood to old age, they said they would be more than willing to help the oldest man and that they would "get his glasses, help him shop, push him in a wheelchair."[3] College students also reflect negativism in our attitudes toward aging.

When asked to compare ideal and real older people with ideal and real middle-aged people, college students consistently rated the older adults in less positive terms, saying they were more dependent and less effective than middle-aged people.[4] Agist attitudes seem intractable, omnipresent. Yet the contradictions between our public attitudes and private actions toward older people offer much hope.

LOOKING AT ONE'S OWN AGING

Most young people do not think about old age. It is pushed into the back of the mind, where it becomes one of the "some day, when I . . ." thoughts to be completed at a much later date. Yet the feelings that we have about our own aging process and our own old age play a large part in determining whether or not we want to work with older people. Most importantly, this attitude has a direct bearing on how effectively we work with the older person. Workers in the field of aging usually agree that it is this interaction between the client and worker that is most related to beneficial change or potential "cure." Those of us who have a positive, accepting view of our own aging are more able to offer compassion, empathy, concern, and appropriate support to our clients; the others communicate their own anxieties, fears, and overconcerns of aging, no matter how well they attempt to mask their feelings. Fearing one's own aging, and working face to face each day with aging people, seems a less than ideal working condition!

Most young students entering the helping professions do not choose to work with the older person. Wilensky and Barmack designed a behavior preference questionnaire to assess the attitudes of clinical psychology doctoral students toward working with the aging. Responses were received from six universities in the New York City area. The authors report strikingly similar response patterns for all six universities, with greatest preference expressed for working with young adults and a tendency for respondents to avoid working with the elderly.[5]

ATTITUDES AS REFLECTED IN THE MEDIA

The U.S. Senate Special Committee, in its 1981 report, stated:

> Attitudes toward the elderly are formed from early life on. Our media helps [sic] shape these attitudes. When reviewing books written within the last 25 years, depicting elderly persons, the prevailing themes in these writings were fear of death and loss of self-image. The older protagonist was shown as being either passively disengaged, exhibiting intergenerational conflict or holding a Pollyanna-ish concept toward reality. Television fared no better. When the older woman appears in a television play or series, she is more than likely to be hurt or killed before the end of the plot or to fail in her attempt to accomplish. The older man is shown as comic, stubborn, or eccentric. Neither sex is generally portrayed as having romantic inclinations.[6]

DEFENSES AGAINST AGING

In order for an attitude to stay ingrained, it must serve some purpose. What could be the purpose in a society's denial of aging? One possibility may relate to the discrepancy between that which is real and that which is ideal. Idealization is part of our training as children. We had figures that we idealized. Sometimes these were real people and sometimes fictional heroes and heroines in books and movies. The ability to idealize is healthy, but when it also denies reality, it becomes defensive. In the case of aging, idealizing is a defense against that which age suggests: deterioration and the setting of limitations. It is against our own need to be "grandiose." In our grandiosity, we can accomplish anything, be anyone, and certainly live forever.[7] Getting older is then denied, repressed, and shelved. It is not for us. As in the classic, *Lost Horizons*, we become a society that is young forever! Our selves never wrinkle or show any age-related changes. Our ideal has come to life!

In our youth-oriented society all that is new, novel, and fresh is to be desired; being old is equated with loss, illness, and eventual death. Why, then, work with the old? What benefits can be gained by the client and by the worker?

JOINING THE AVANT-GARDE

Those who are aware do not deny their own aging or that of others; yet the battle against agism in our society is a continuous one. Major programs of public education are developing to combat prejudice toward the old and to improve the image of the aging experience in the eyes of the general public, the media, service providers, and the elderly themselves.[8] Any action that helps combat age discrimination is an avant-garde one. People joining these ranks are breaking new ground in creating much-needed, positive changes in our society.

OLD PEOPLE CAN CHANGE

In order to gain satisfaction from working with people, the worker needs to feel that he or she has had an impact on the person seeking help. This positive change in the client helps confirm and reinforce the worker's own sense of effectiveness. Although much of society's projected image of the old person is that he or she is incapable of change or that "it is all organic," those working with the aged, in whatever setting, dispute this. The authors, for example, have seen patients in their 80s and 90s being discharged from an institution as a result of positive changes in their physical and psychological status, attributed (in part) to therapeutic efforts. This may be replicated by noticeable positive changes in those elderly who have come for psychological counseling or psychotherapy. Old people, like the young and middle-aged, can be helped to change if *both* they and the worker believe that this help is possible. This belief may be the most essential step toward promoting change.

QUALITY VERSUS QUANTITY

Though the older person is closer to the end of life than the younger, the worker must feel that helping someone live out the rest of his or her years satisfactorily is a most worthwhile endeavor, even if those years are limited in number. The quality of a life's experience cannot be measured in the same way as its quantity; numbers of years may have little to do with satisfactions in living. The only possible way to help measure relieving another person's human suffering or to help make life better for him or her is in terms of one's own internalized value system; that is, a sense of one's own feelings of accomplishment and heightened self-esteem through reaching out and offering assistance to another. The quality of this experience, regardless of its time span, will then be felt and appreciated, not only by the older person, but also by the worker. Only this form of mutuality leads to positive change in both.

OLD PEOPLE APPRECIATE HELP

The older population is often a population in need. Experiencing physical and psychosocial declines, the older person is often in need of some kind of help. This dependence may reflect itself in the depth and intensity of appreciation extended to the worker, the one who is "there for me." When offered assistance, the client's first comment may be, "Why bother with me when there are younger people around to help?" This is undoubtedly a reflection on society's values, which focus attention on the young. If, however, a worker can go beyond this overt verbalization and initial resistance and can sincerely reach out to help, gratitude is deep. This acts as a positive reinforcer that deepens one's own sense of self-worth as well as professional and personal competence. Being thanked or appreciated by the client confirms that one is wanted and needed. In addition, the experience of change in the client reconfirms the worker's belief that life at any stage involves continued growth and development.

PRACTICAL CONSIDERATIONS

It is common knowledge that all Americans are living longer, that longevity is on the increase. According to the 1980 census, there are 25.5 million people over age 65 residing in the United States; this represents 11.3 percent of the U.S. population. By the year 2000, there will be 32 million individuals aged 65 and over in the United States, or 12 percent of the population, while projections for the year 2030 indicate that there will be about 55 million elderly.[9] By that time, the overall 65-and-over population will double, while the 85-and-over population will *triple*.[10]

The need for persons who work in the field of aging is therefore also on the rise. One needs only to look at recent data on geriatric medicine to realize this. For example, between the years 1982 and 1984, the American Academy of Family Physicians developed particular core curricula guidelines dealing specifically with aging and the care of the aged for family practice residents. In addition, in 1982, a standing committee was formed by the Committee on Geriatric Rehabilitation of the American Academy of Physical Medicine and Rehabilitation. In terms of increased medical education in aging, it is suggested that there be "continual updating of standards of accreditation . . . to allow for better training in geriatric medicine." Geriatric medicine will be included at each level of physicians' training in the future.[11]

The field of aging, therefore, still offers work opportunities, not only for physicians, but for all those involved in the care of older people. A look at the employment section of any newspaper confirms this. "Arming" oneself with skills and insights for working with this age group appears consistent with needed services and societal trends. The aged are here to stay, and they are here to stay longer. We should be prepared to work with them.

YOUR OWN QUALITIES AND GROWTH EXPERIENCE

There are still relatively few data on the qualities needed to make one effective in working with the older person. In a study by Conte, Weiner, Plutchik, Bennett, and White seeking to discriminate between nurses' aides considered by their supervisors to be successful or unsuccessful in working with older patients, the authors found that successful aides ranked higher on qualities of patience, acceptance, flexibility, tolerance, and respect.[12] Certain factors may appear self-evident, such as that the older person is usually slower responding and therefore requires more time to complete a task. Similarly, not accepted as a full citizen by a society geared to the young, the older person does best with a worker/therapist who shows a good degree of acceptance and respect for his or her many years of living. In addition, if the worker has flexibility of style, this can act as a modifier toward what may be perceived negatively as the older person's "rigidity" but which, upon closer examination, is often a necessary need for preserving and clinging tightly to that which is familiar.

How then does one evaluate the extent of these qualities in oneself? The answer may be only by trying to get in touch with the feelings one has toward working with the older adult, by reflecting upon, examining, and accepting these feelings, whatever they may be. The adage of being true to oneself could not be more apt!

If one does conclude that he or she is motivated to work with the aging person, the satisfactions are found to be many. Primary are satisfactions related to the worker's own growth experience. Those who work in the field of psychotherapy, in particular, have written much on the interaction between client and therapist. Emphasis is placed on the fact that much of the client's improvement is contingent on the relationship with "a new object," the therapist.[13] Change can also come about in the worker/therapist if he or she is in tune, not only with the client's world, but also his or her own. By interactions with the client, a worker can become a more integrated, better functioning, better feeling person. This may come about partially through empathic understanding and mutual identifications. The older client may see in the younger worker both his or her own youthful past and possibilities for the future; the worker, often younger, may see in the client portions of his or her own aging. In this way each is able to foresee and possibly play out a trial fantasy for a phase of one's own future existence. This integration of past and present with the future provides both client and worker with a most viable frame of reference for living and may serve as the basis for optimal growth experiences.

REFERENCE NOTES

1. Weiner, M. B., Teresi, J., & Streich, C. *Old people are a burden, but not my parents*. Englewood Cliffs, N.J.: Prentice-Hall, Inc. 1983.
2. Seefeldt, C., Jantz, R., Galper, A., & Serock, K. Using pictures to explore children's attitudes toward the elderly. *The Gerontologist*, 1977, *17*(6), 506–509.
3. Weinberger, A. Stereotyping of the elderly. *Research on Aging*, 1979, *1*(1), 113–136.
4. Sherman, N., & Gold, J. Perceptions of ideal and typical middle and old age. *International Journal of Aging and Human Development*, 1978, 67–73.
5. Wilensky, H., & Barmack, J. Interests of doctoral students in clinical psychology in work with older adults. *Journal of Gerontology*, 1966, *21*, 410–414.
6. U.S. Senate Special Committee on Aging. *Developments in aging*, 1981. Vol. 1, Special Research 45, March 3, 1981. Washington, D.C., February, 1982.
7. White, M. T., & Weiner, M. B. *The theory and practice of self psychology*. New York: Brunner/Mazel, 1986.
8. The Reports of The President's Commission on Mental Health: Task Panel on the Elderly. *Mental health and the elderly, recommendations for action*. U.S. Dept. of Health, Education and Welfare, DHEW Publication No. (OHDS) 80-20960, 1979, p. 93.
9. U.S. Senate Special Committee on Aging, 1982.
10. U.S. Bureau of the Census. *U.S. Census*, 1980.
11. Steel, K. Geriatric medicine is coming of age. *The Gerontologist*, 1984, *24*(4), 367–372.
12. Conte, H., Weiner, M. B., & Plutchik, R., et al. *Selecting successful workers with aged persons: An empirical investigation*. Paper presented at the 46th annual meeting of the Eastern Psychological Association, New York, 1975.
13. Loewald, H. W. On the therapeutic action of psycho-analysis. *International Journal of Psychoanalysis*, 1960, *41*, 16–33.

2

Physiological Aging

Although we all begin the aging process at conception, the point at which we classify ourselves, or find ourselves classified by society, as being "old" can vary tremendously. Pinpointing the aged population depends on, and involves, an understanding of the various ways in which the aging process is conceptualized. Aging may be narrowly viewed in terms of particular physical characteristics and biological processes, or it may be more broadly viewed from social, cultural, legal, psychological, or experiential perspectives. More often than not, all of the above perspectives, whether broad or narrow, have a place in defining the category "aged." Indeed, it is only through understanding the interrelationships among the various perspectives that we can truly comprehend what is meant by the concept "growing old." In this and the following chapter, we discuss some of the ways of defining who the aged are and consider issues relevant to each definition, as well as to their integration.

What are the signs of aging? What is normal aging? Are there basic physiological processes that change with age in the absence of disease? What limits the length of human life? These are some of the critical issues involved in defining *who the aged are* in biological terms.

SIGNS OF AGING

Perhaps the most apparent signs of aging involve the appearance of changes in a person's physical characteristics. The gradual emergence of graying hair and skin wrinkles, the loss of teeth, poor eyesight, decreased hearing acuity, and various postural changes are all signs that seem to give clear and unequivocal indications of age. Such changes, however, are not directly correlated with any specific chronological age but are subject to wide individual differences.[1]

To many, chronological age (our actual age in years) is the principal sign of old age. It is common in the American culture to consider anyone who has reached the age of 65 as "old." Although chronological age is a good general indicator of physical abilities, it leaves a lot to be desired as a basis for making assumptions about any particular individual's physical health or sense of psychological well-being. The person who looks old may not feel old or, for that matter, even be old in chronological terms. On the other hand, someone whose physical appearance indicates a "youthful" 65 may feel very depressed about his or her chronological age.

There is little doubt that the relationship between general functioning and chronological age is strongly modified by individual differences. Although there is an abundance of research showing that the most characteristic sign of advanced chronological age is a decline in the speed of both mental and physical functioning, a number of exceptions to this generalization have been observed. Jarvik, for example, repeatedly tested one older female during a 20-year period (from age 60 to 80) and reported no decline in scores on a tapping test.[2] Research with elderly drivers showed that many of them had reaction times comparable to those of young drivers, although *on the average* they were slower.[3]

Similarly, Botwinick and Thompson observed no differences in reaction times between 68- to 86-year-old males and a group of males aged 18 to 22 who were not particularly athletic. These researchers suggest that such extrinsic factors as amount of daily exercise, rather than decrements associated with chronological age, could (in part) account for observed similarities or differences in reaction times between age groups.[4] In fact, the extent of individual differences is so great that many older subjects perform more quickly than younger subjects in laboratory reaction-time experiments.[5]

NORMAL AGING AND DISEASE STATES

One difficulty in describing the process of *normal aging* from a biological perspective is that many of the physical and biological changes observed with increasing age may be the results of disease states related to age rather than to the aging process itself. Although research shows that human cells grown in laboratory cultures seem to have a limited capacity to duplicate, and that individuals experience a decline in integrated body functions at the rate of approximately 1 percent per year, many scientists continue to believe that no one really dies of "old age."[6] Rather, death is caused by specific diseases or disorders that are in some way correlated with old age—that is, aging may be a process that increases the probability of disease.[7]

The problem of clearly distinguishing between "abnormal" disorders that can be treated medically or psychologically, and changes that are inevitable as a result of age, is a long-standing one. If we look at assumptions of old age throughout history, we can see that the process of normal aging has often been confused with the process of disease and decline. Since many of the program designs and activities suggested for working with or rehabilitating the aged are based on assumptions about what might be expected from the "normal aged," it becomes extremely important to distinguish between the biases handed down through history and factual material about the aging process. In this framework, let us now look at some of the theories of normal aging offered throughout the past and see how these theories might affect current program ideals and goals.

THEORIES OF NORMAL AGING FROM THE PAST

Since ancient times, the concept of aging as an inevitable and normal process of decline, similar to that of a disease state, has been considered the most basic explanation for growing old. Perhaps this is because of the historical connection between the emergence of medical science and the study of aging.[8] For example, one of the earliest biologically oriented theories of aging was generated by Hippocrates, the Greek philosopher considered the father of modern medicine. He believed that old age was caused by the progressive imbalance in what was then thought of as the four basic body substances—blood, phlegm, choler, and black choler. Interestingly, these imbalances were also thought to be the cause of sickness. It seems clear that Hippocrates tended to view the process of aging as being caused by the same factors as illness. The Greek philosopher–scientist was also the first to express the stages of human development in terms of the four seasons, with old age, as we might expect, relegated to winter.[9] The winter analogy remains a popular symbol today and underlies the biologically oriented view of the inevitability of aging as being equal to decline. During the Middle Ages, old age was also generally looked upon as an incurable disease, and even during the Renaissance, the growth of interest in human anatomy and science in general did not seem to greatly change basic conceptions of the aging process.[10]

Since the Renaissance, many physical and biological theories of aging have been generated. Perhaps two of the most significant can be termed the *wear-and-tear theory* and the *declining-energy theory*. As with all theories, these two tend to be based on the prevailing philosophical conception of man at a particular point in the historical development of a culture. In terms of the aging process, this means that *how* aging is understood is in part dependent on *what* we believe is responsible for human functioning. By studying some of these prevailing philosophical conceptions, we can perhaps understand the rationale behind various programs, goals, and ideals developed for working with the aged.

Wear-and-Tear Theory: Man as a Machine

Although the viewpoint that a human is essentially similar to a complex mechanical device whose parts are replaceable can be traced back to classical times—such as when Aristotle noted that an old man needed only the eye of a young man in order to look like a young man[11]—the concept of *man as a machine* has continued to be important throughout history. This concept seems to have gained popularity especially during the 18th and 19th centuries with the emergence of the philosophical school of rationalism. Believing that the mind and body were separate, Descartes argued that the body functions operated essentially like a complex machine.[12] In the field of medicine, this sort of thinking had great influence on a group of scientists called *iatrophysicists*.

Iatrophysics, a school of medicine especially popular in the 18th century, attempted to combine the concepts of mechanical physics with medicine. Specifically, scientists of this school tried to explain both disease processes and activities of the body in terms of physics instead of chemistry. To iatrophysicists, the process of normal aging occurred as a result of body deterioration, just as a machine wears out when it has been used for too long.[13]

This wear-and-tear theory remains popular today. To note its continuing impact, we have only to think of the hope many people have that organ transplants can ensure longevity by replacing "the old, used-up parts of the body" with new, functional ones. Unfortunately, the "spare-parts" concept inherent in such a theory does not seem plausible as a method for increasing the life span. It appears that specific organ transplants do not affect the apparent decline with age in the efficiency of complex homeostatic mechanisms or in the process of cellular aging.[14]

Implications of the Wear-and-Tear Theory. From a social point of view, we believe that the continuing impact of the wear-and-tear theory can still be observed as a subtle influence on the program goals and ideals of those working with the aged. Machines are things of motion; they function best when kept running at a steady pace. Inactivity or disuse can lead to rust and the need for replacement. When such thinking is translated into life-style values, it is reflective of the prevailing American ethic, "keep active, keep busy, keep in motion."

It was perhaps no accidental finding when a recent sociological survey revealed a 73-year-old man as saying that his main goal in life is to "keep active—I want to wear out, not rust out."[15] This fear of "rusting," of the machine wearing down, may be a major psychological issue for many older Americans. The overidentification with machine-type attributes may, in turn, lead to an overemphasis on compulsive activity or "doing" patterns and to a de-emphasis on the value of contemplation, leisure, or "being" states. Social scientists have indicated that Americans do not, as a rule, take easily (or readily) to leisure when it is made available in the form of retirement.[16]

Critiques by Eastern (e.g., Indian) psychiatric viewpoints of American- and Western-style therapies include the notion that Americans tend not to enjoy the simple experience of "being" with each other but feel that they must "get or achieve something" out of doing things with each other.[17] Such notions are buried deep in the American ethic of the need for achievement. When combined with an identification with mechanistic analogies, they often form the basis for program goals and ideals that roughly follow the dictates of the *activity theory*.

Basically, this theory involves the notion that "if you keep busy, you stay healthy." As we shall see in Part III, which deals with the community aged, such thinking may lead to activity programs in which *what* old people keep busy *with* is considered less important than the *mere activity* of keeping busy. Although certainly of some benefit, when uncritically accepted, the attitude that people should be kept busy can lead workers and programmers to erroneously overfocus on the *number* of activities, with diminishing concern for the *quality* of the activities. This can also lead to a diminished concern with the quality of the relationships engendered by a program, in deference to a "numbers count" attitude. Quantity of social acquaintances does not necessarily mean good quality of friendship experiences.

The Declining-Energy Theory: Human Beings as Having Limited Vitality

The concept of humans as biological energy systems, like dry cell batteries that cannot be recharged, is implicit in various theories of aging. For example, aging has been thought of as a progressive decline of vigor and resistance with the passage of time or as a decline in physiological competence that both increases and intensifies the effects of various forms of environmental stress.[18,19] Two important notions about the aging process emerge from the following definitions:

1. Aging implies a decline in either energy or vigor.
2. This decline results in a lower ability to deal with outside forces (lessened resistance to and tolerance of environmental stress).

The idea that aging implies some sort of innate energy decline is partially derived from the philosophy of *vitalism*. The vitalists were early biologists and philosophers who were not content with the purely physical theories of life popular during the middle ages. In particular, they believed that life was at least in some part self-determining instead of mechanistically determined, and they therefore postulated the existence of an energy source that was nonphysical. The existence of this nonphysical energy source, or *vital principle,* was thought to "use" the physical apparatus of the body (such as the nerves, muscles, and specialized organs) as a means to act on the natural world.[20] The vitalistic assumption indicates that the gradual loss of this energy over time, and its ultimate disappearance, is what brings about old age and eventually death.[21] It is interesting to note that a similar notion was implicit in Freud's theory of libido—an instinctual energy that conceivably dissipates with age.[22]

Variations on the idea of declining energy as an explanation for the process of aging have not been confined to Western European thinking. Holmberg noted that various Andean tribal groups have the following belief on aging:

> . . . the human organism has in its constitution a given number of ounces of earth. The quantity, although fixed for the individual, varies from person to person. Some have more, others less. The existence of strong and weak people, in fact, is explained on the basis that some people have more earth in their constitutions than others. Those having the greatest amount are also those who show the greatest physical resistance on such occasions as drinking feasts and religious festivals, which are popular and widespread institutions in the Andes.[23]

Although never proven, assumptions about aging that are related to or derived from vitalistic notions have maintained their appeal over many centuries. In modern times, they exemplify the battery analogy of man—that we have a fixed amount of energy, which we use up (or run out of) over time.

Implications of the Declining-Energy Theory. The belief that people have a limited amount of vitality that dissipates with age may still continue to exert influences on both theories of aging and practices of working with the aged. Those working with the aged might tend to believe that old people prefer to *disengage* from society, that they prefer to be left alone to reminisce or reflect on the past instead of engaging in face-to-face interaction in the environment. Cumming and Henry, for example, have proposed a formalized *disengagement theory of aging* based on data obtained from a sample of Kansas City elderly.[24] In their sample, they found that chronological aging was accompanied by a steady decline in social interaction, ego, and energy involvement in the social environment and by a decline in role activity.

From these and related data, it has been proposed that normal successful aging involves a mutual disengagement between individual and society. The disengagement theory implies that the sources of psychological well-being in old age are substantially different from those of middle age, which are assumed to be more dependent on high levels of social activity and social–interpersonal interaction.[25]

The disengagement theory encourages those who work with the aged to believe that much interest and involvement in the "outer world" should not be expected of old people. This sort of thinking can subtly influence policy and program goals to de-emphasize remotivational-type programs, which encourage continued exploration and interest in the environment. Such thinking may also serve as a rationalization to maintain forced retirement policies and to discourage retraining those who are already retired.

Further research on the disengagement theory seems to indicate that the process of normal psychologically successful aging is not solely related to the need for a timely mutual disengagement of the individual and the society. Instead, it is strongly determined and moderated by individual personality characteristics.[26] Neugarten, Havighurst, and Tobin note:

> People, as they grow old, seem to be neither at the mercy of the social environment nor at the mercy of some set of intrinsic processes—in either instance, inexorable changes that they cannot influence. On the contrary, the individual seems to continue to make his own "impress" upon the wide range of social and biological changes. He continues to exercise choice and to select from the environment in accordance with his own long-established needs. He ages according to a pattern that has a long history, and that maintains itself, with adaptation, to the end of life.[27]

We believe that it is important for those who work with, or create programs for, the aged to be sensitive to the individual characteristics of the elderly.

DISTINGUISHING BETWEEN NORMAL AGING AND DISEASE STATES IN RECENT TIMES

As we have seen, the problem of clearly distinguishing between abnormal disorders to be treated and changes that are "inevitable" as a result of age has been a long-standing one throughout history. The ability to draw such clear-cut distinctions still remains a difficult task.

The problem of correctly assessing age differences in blood pressure is one simple example of the current difficulty in discriminating between disease states and the normal aging process. As we grow older, measurements of diastolic, and particularly systolic, blood pressure tend to be higher than when we were younger. Hypertension, which is associated with high blood pressure, is also a physical sign of a number of serious diseases that can be medically treated. When faced with these facts, health professionals have to decide whether observed high blood pressure in an older individual should be medically treated or considered normal. Underlying such a decision is the problem of deciding whether standards of normality for blood pressure should be adjusted for age.[28] On this and related issues, Bierman and Hazzard note:

> Blood pressure is only one of the many examples of the principle that the change in organ function with age may be indistinguishable in magnitude, direction, and character from the change in function which occurs in well-defined disease states. Tests of pulmonary or renal function clearly demonstrate progressive decrements with increasing age which resemble the common chronic pulmonary and renal diseases. In these instances, however, where therapy [medical treatment] is by *no* means as effective or as readily evaluated as in the hypertensive diseases, and where the measurements themselves are not as simple to perform, the relation of age change to disease has *not* become as pressing a problem. [However, let us] . . . consider also the condition of prostatism. Here, our ability to quantitate the change with age [or disease?] is *poor* indeed and the therapy, surgery, not one to be undertaken *lightly*. . . . The point to be made by these examples is that the conditions of a particular historical moment strongly influence the physician's view toward aging and disease.[29]

We can see that, even today, it is not a simple matter to clearly distinguish the aging process from the process of disease.

SOME BASIC PHYSIOLOGICAL PROCESSES THAT CHANGE WITH AGE IN THE ABSENCE OF DISEASE

Homeostasis

Although we may not be able to specify the exact causes of aging, we can describe various changes that seem to occur along with age. For example, the body's ability to regulate levels of blood pH, blood sugar, and pulse rate under various and changing conditions seems to decline with age. In general, research shows that there is almost a linear decline of approximately 1 percent per year in most integrated body functions in adult life.[30] Despite these facts, it also has been shown that old people maintain basic homeostatic balances (the way the body stabilizes its physiological functioning) as efficiently as younger persons under resting conditions. What seems to be problematical is that advanced age greatly impairs the body's capacity to favorably readjust internal functioning after experiencing stressful circumstances.[31] This decline in ability to maintain a proper homeostatic balance in the face of stress is one of the major problems of normal aging. Some scientists, for example, have estimated that, if we kept the same resistance and resilience to stress throughout our life span that we had at age 12, half of us alive today could expect to live another 700 years.[32]

The likelihood that older people react more severely to stress than do younger people carries implications for programming and for working with the aged. Techniques used in working with the aged should perhaps take into account the "excitatory potential" or stress of the social and physical environments. For example, we have elsewhere outlined the various problem source areas and stresses to which older people are especially vulnerable. Briefly summarized, these involve decreases in sensory capacities and physical mobility, loss of status and shrinkage of roles, various psychological life crises engendered by realization of the loss of youth, and philosophical crises induced by thoughts about the general meaning of life. The stresses to which the aged are susceptible can therefore come from many sources. "Best fit" models of treatment should take into account the source of each particular stress, as well as how the individual aged person copes with each stress.

Cell and Tissue Aging

Until recently, the theory that aging involves the progressive loss of cells was widely accepted. Cell loss was thought to be responsible for decreased muscular strength, impairment of brain functioning, and other symptoms of old age. The greatest loss of cells in humans seems to occur in the brain, skeletal muscles, and kidneys, with some loss found in the liver.[33] Although still of some importance, cell loss is not currently considered a crucial factor in normal aging.

In opposition to the decreasing importance of cell loss as a factor in aging, there is a strong controversy about the effects of cellular aging. One of the basic issues here is whether or not human cells have a finite life span. One fascinating group of findings reported by Hayflick seems to indicate that cells *do* have a definite life span. He reports that cells grown in laboratory cultures die out after 50 doublings.[34] Bierman and Hazzard also indicate that human cells grown in tissue culture do not divide indefinitely but instead show a decreasing capacity for finite division with age. They note that cells taken from a human embryo divide about 50 times in culture, while those taken from a 20-year-old duplicate about 30 times. In comparison, cells obtained from older donors divide about 20 times.[35] The propensity for cells to be limited by a finite number of duplications appears to occur across animal species. For example, comparison of aging of normal cells derived from different animal species also shows that considerable differences exist between species, with man being second to the Galapagos tortoise. Table 2–1 summarizes the available data on cross-species differences.

Does all of this mean that the mechanism for aging is to be found in the finiteness of cell duplication? The answer is not clear but what seems certain is that "conditions have yet to be found that will permit normal cell populations to replicate indefinitely."[36] Hayflick goes on to say that this failure of cell replication could be changed by the finding of some nutritional or growth factor. This has not been found. He concludes that normal cells, whether "cultured in vitro or serially transplanted in vivo, ultimately incur physiological decrements and die." This, he sug-

TABLE 2–1. THE FINITE LIFETIME OF CULTURED NORMAL EMBRYONIC HUMAN AND ANIMAL FIBROBLASTS

Species	Range of Population Doublings for Cultured Normal Embryo Fibroblasts (Cells)	Mean Maximum Life Span in Years
Galapagos tortoise	90–125	175 (?)
Man	40–60	110
Mink	30–34	10
Chicken	15–35	30 (?)
Mouse	14–28	3.5

Adapted from Hayflick, L. Why grow old? The Stanford Magazine, *1975,* 3, *36–43.*

gests, may be defined as aging or "differentiation to death," a task that he assigns to semanticists rather than biologists! To date, it seems clear that "since most animal species have a specific life span, normal somatic cells composing their tissues obviously die as well."[37]

Aging at the Molecular Level

There are some who believe that the aging process may be the result of the accumulation of "errors" in "the genetic matrix which generates the many physiochemical systems supporting cell biosynthesis and homeostatic regulation."[38] Specifically, it seems that problems arise over time in the genetically programmed DNA–RNA enzyme protein synthesis necessary for the proper functioning of cells. DNA (deoxyribonucleic acid) determines the formation of RNA (ribonucleic acid), which in turn produces enzymes involved in cellular functioning. The errors that might occur include mutations, cross-linkages, incorrect transcription (in the formation of RNA and DNA), etc. All of these factors can create *creeping error* in the cell system and contribute to the production of *anamolous* protein.[39] Such cumulative errors may be a major source of changes leading to senescence.[40]

Unfortunately, scientists disagree on why these changes occur. There are those who argue that such changes are evolutionary while others believe that these problems "are essentially random events that accumulate with age until the cell itself becomes defective."[41]

Autoimmunity and Accumulation of Metabolic Waste

Various other theories on the aging process have been proposed. One involves the notion that aging occurs because cells are slowly poisoned by metabolic waste products that accumulate over time. Another theory proposes that over time the body builds up immunity to its own tissues through the production of autoimmune antibodies. This process would theoretically lead to cell dysfunction and death. These theories are generally unproven, however, and are considered symptoms rather than causes of aging.[42]

THE GOOD NEWS FROM THE BRAIN

Although human beings seem to be programmed for a finite, though increasing, life span, the good news is that the brain continues to grow into old age. Once thought to be fixed by late childhood, new evidence shows that "even in old age the cells of the cerebral cortex respond to an enriched environment by forging new connections to other cells."[43] The fact that there is such neural flexibility in old age is astonishing and implies to workers in the field of aging and to society in general that we can help create the enriched environment that can spur this growth.

REFERENCE NOTES

1. Jarvik, L. F. Thoughts on the psychobiology of aging. *American Psychologist*, 1975, *30*, 576–583.
2. Ibid.
3. Giantucco, D. T., Ramm, D., & Erwin, C. W. The elderly driver and ex-driver. In E. Palmore (Ed.), *Normal aging II*. Durham, N.C.: Duke University Press, 1974, pp. 173–179.
4. Botwinick, J., & Thompson, L. W. Cardiac functioning and reaction time in relation to age. *Journal of Genetic Psychology*, 1971, *119*, 127–132.
5. Botwinick, J. *Aging and behavior*. New York: Springer, 1984.
6. Hayflick, L. Aging under glass. *Experimental Gerontology*, 1970, *5*, 291–304.
7. Bierman, E. L., & Hazzard, W. R. Biology of Aging. In D. W. Smith & E. L. Bierman (Eds.), *The biologic ages of man, from conception through old age*. Philadelphia: Saunders, 1973.
8. de Beauvoir, S. *The coming of age*. New York: G.P. Putnam's Sons, 1972.
9. Ibid.
10. Ibid.
11. Zilboorg, G. A. *A history of medical psychology*. New York: W.W. Norton and Co., 1941.
12. Kohler, W. *The task of gestalt psychology*. Princeton, N.J.: Princeton University Press, 1969.
13. de Beauvoir, *The coming of age*.
14. Kimmel, D. C. *Adulthood and aging*. New York: Wiley, 1974.
15. Bengston, V. L. *The social psychology of aging*. New York: Bobbs-Merrill, 1973, p. 6.
16. Hooker, K., & Ventis, D. G. Work ethic, daily activities and retirement satisfaction. *Journal of Gerontology*, 1984, *39*(4), 478–484.
17. Pande, S. K. The mystique of "western" psychotherapy: An eastern interpretation. *The Journal of Nervous and Mental Disease*, 1968, *146*, 425–432.
18. Bierman & Hazzard, *Biology of aging*.
19. Timiras, P. S. *Developmental physiology and aging*. New York: Macmillan, 1972.
20. Langer, S. K. *Mind: An essay on human feeling*. Baltimore: The Johns Hopkins Press, 1967.
21. de Beauvoir, *The coming of age*.
22. Freud, S. *An outline of psycho-analysis*. New York: W.W. Norton and Co., 1969.
23. Holmberg, A. R. Age in the Andes. In R. W. Kleemeir (Ed.), *Aging and leisure*. New York: Oxford University Press, 1961, pp. 86–87.

24. Cumming, E., & Henry, W. E. *Growing old: The process of disengagement*. New York: Basic Books, 1961.
25. Bengston, *The social psychology of aging*.
26. Neugarten, B. L., Havighurst, R. J., & Tobin, S. S. Personality and patterns of aging. In B. L. Neugarten (Ed.), *Middle age and aging*. Chicago: The University of Chicago Press, 1968.
27. Ibid., p. 177.
28. Bierman, E. L. & Hazzard, W. R. Old age, including death and dying. In D. W. Smith & E. L. Bierman (Eds.), *The biologic ages of man, from conception through old age*, Philadelphia: Saunders, 1973.
29. Ibid., pp. 174–175.
30. Ibid.
31. Kimmel, *Adulthood and aging*.
32. Bierman & Hazzard, *Biology of aging*.
33. Jarvik, L. F., & Cohen, D. A biobehavioral approach to intellectual changes with aging. In C. Eisdorfer, & M. P. Lawton (Eds.), *The psychology of adult development and aging*. Washington D.C.: American Psychological Association, 1973.
34. Hayflick, L. Why grow old? *The Stanford Magazine*, 1975, *3*, 36–43.
35. Bierman & Hazzard, *Biology of aging*.
36. Hayflick, L. Cell aging. In C. Eisdorfer, et al. (Eds.), *Annual review of gerontology and geriatrics*. New York: Springer, 1980.
37. Ibid.
38. Jarvik & Cohen. A biobehavioral approach to intellectual changes with aging, p. 234.
39. Ibid.
40. Orgel, L. E. The maintenance of the accuracy of protein synthesis and its relevance to aging. *Proceedings of the National Academy of Sciences*, 1963, *49*, 517–521.
41. Kimmel, *Adulthood and aging*, p. 355.
42. Ibid.
43. Science Times, *N.Y. Times*, June 30, 1985, p. C1.

3

Psychological Aging

ASPECTS OF NORMAL PERSONALITY DEVELOPMENT IN OLD AGE

Although it has been generally acknowledged throughout history that people continue to develop and change as they grow older, relatively little psychological data on this phase of the life cycle were systematically presented before the early 20th century. Until the 1920s, the comprehension of personality in later life had not moved much beyond Shakespeare's classic statement on the seven ages of man:

> All the world's a stage,
> And all the men and women merely players;
> They have their exits and their entrances,
> And one man in his time plays many parts,
> His acts being seven ages. At first the infant. . .
> Then the whining schoolboy. . .
> Creeping like a snail,
>   Unwillingly to school. And then the lover,
> Sighing like a furnace. . .
> Then a soldier,
> Full of strange oaths and bearded like the pard,
> Jealous in honor, sudden and quick in quarrel,
> Seeking the bubble reputation,
> Even in the cannon's mouth. And then the justice. . .
> With eyes severe and beard of formal cut,
> Full of wise saws and modern instances. . .
>   The sixth age shifts
> Into the lean and slippered pantaloon,
> With spectacles on nose and pouch on side;

His youthful hose, well saved, a world too wide
For his shrunk shank, and his big manly voice,
Turning again toward childish treble, pipes
And whistles in his sound. Last scene of all,
That ends this strange eventful history,
Is second childishness and mere oblivion,
Sans teeth, sans eyes, sans taste, sans everything.

As You Like It

Shakespeare's belief that old age was equivalent to an empty "second childishness and mere oblivion" may still be considered true by some of those working with the aged because of the nature of some of the simple activity programs available to many of our senior citizens. Fortunately, there seems to be more to old age than Shakespeare would have us believe. In this light, we consider some of the prominent theories and concepts that relate to personality development in later life.

THE TWO MAJOR THEMES

Gerontology is dominated by two themes that usually belong to theology and philosophy. One of these involves the question of man's immortality. Are we mortal or potentially immortal? The other theme has to do with our beliefs about the universe and life's processes in relation to aging. Is our world to be considered good or evil? These themes are part of every theory (whether or not they are obvious), much as all gerontologists, in their professional activities, are influenced by their own views about aging and death.[1]

Behavior is an outgrowth of personality. While behavior changes with age, can we assume that this implies a change in personality? Most theorists say "no." They admit that there may be dramatic changes in later-life behaviors, so that, for example, an older person may be more interested in walking or gardening than in playing an active sport (though there are many older marathon runners!), but these changes "do not amount to change in personality."[2] It is usually accepted that there are few, if any, behavioral changes with age. "Personality is stable, not changing, during adulthood."[3]

STAGE THEORIES

Stage theories are as the word implies: Life's development is a succession of stages; each is a step one climbs in reaching a particular goal. Once a stage has been passed, there is no going backwards. Each stage is a separate entity and is different from the ones preceding or following it.

While most stage theories cover the earlier years (infancy, young childhood, late childhood, and adolescence), few cover the middle years and continue to old age. Yet stage theories are helpful, in that they describe general developmental patterns; some, as we shall see, go on to describe patterns in the later years.

Buhler: Self-Fulfillment and Goals in Later Life

The Viennese psychologist Charlotte Buhler was one of the first researchers to actually gather data on issues faced in old age. She collected life histories in autobiographical form from elderly people.[4] In the present context, Buhler's principal contribution was the suggestion that the life span can be divided into various phases or stages that do not completely parallel (but rather, are similar to) the biological life course of growth, stability, and decline. Implicit in her findings were the notions that mental abilities such as intelligence do not decline as rapidly as physical capacities and that old age may be a time for continued goal development and concerns about self-fulfillment. Interviews with older people showed that fulfillment in old age often involved the following four major considerations:

1. *The aspect of luck.* Fulfilled people almost always seem to mention that their life involved meeting the right persons or being at the right place at the right time. Religious persons view this as the work of God. Unfulfilled people view their life as marked by bad luck.
2. *Feelings about the realization of one's potentialities.* Fulfilled people note that "I did most of what I wanted to do," or "I did what was right for me." Unfulfilled people display the opposite feelings.
3. *The aspect of accomplishment.* Whether there is the feeling that there is "something to show" for one's past life is a major contributing factor to satisfaction or dissatisfaction in later life.
4. *Moral evaluation.* Individuals who seem fulfilled tend to emphasize that they have "lived right"; this is meant in terms of their religious or moral convictions. Fulfilled people seem to emphasize that they have dedicated themselves to some highly valued objective in family relations, made progress in some important field of endeavor, or given their support to various social groups.[5]

In general, Buhler believed that personality-oriented suggestions about the achievement of fulfillment in later life were more critical for psychological adjustment in old age than either biological decline or the experiences of insecurity engendered by social losses.

Jung: The Process of Individuation in Later Life

C. G. Jung was one of the first psychiatrists to break from total agreement with Freudian theory. The emphasis that Freud placed on the early years of life dissatisfied Jung, who believed that human life involves a continual series of *metamorphoses,* changes in personality orientation, through which the process of *individuation* can be achieved.[6] One goal of the individuation process is the unification of personality. Simply stated, Jung viewed the personality as being made up of various psychic components, such as the anima and animus (male and female traits) and the shadow (ignored aspects of the self). Although Jung did view old age as a period of complete dependence on others and, in some respects, as a stage similar to childhood, he had much to say about personality changes specific to old age.[7]

Perhaps the principal contribution made by Jung to the personality of old age was his postulation of changes in the process of psychic organization of the self. This process involved a tendency for the personality to change in the direction of the opposite sex. Thus, he believed that the female component (anima) in older men became more prominent and that women became more masculine in their psychological orientation as they aged.

Interestingly, cross-cultural research concerned with age changes in the psychological stances of both men and women seem to uphold Jung's earlier clinically derived notions. Guttman, for example, notes that, in contrast to younger men, older men are less aggressive, more affiliative, more interested in love than in power, more aesthetic, less businesslike, and more sensitive to the importance of incidental pleasures. He also states that older men turn toward a psychology of "diffuse sensuality"; that is, they become particularly interested in food, pleasant sights and sounds, and human associations. Guttman further reports that studies across a wide range of cultures show that women age psychologically in the opposite direction of men. That is, they become more aggressive, less sentimental, and more domineering.[8]

These results are not related to specific individuals, but they do describe general trends based on group data. Such psychological sex role changes might indeed take their toll on married couples in later life if husband and wife do not understand this process.

Although Jung considered the natural end in life to be wisdom rather than senility, he believed that the aged individual could only achieve such wisdom by not competing with the youth of society or clinging to the past. Jung appears to have strongly believed that the perpetuation of pseudo-youthful images by the aged in Western societies was deplorable in comparison to the dignity accorded to elders observed in certain anthropological tribal studies.[9] Rather than clinging to the past or competing with youth, Jung maintained that the old person must not deny his or her current reality and that death should not be "a peril to shrink from . . . [for] . . . an old man who cannot bid farewell to life appears as feeble and sickly as a young man who is unable to embrace it."[10]

Jung further suggests that, as the individual ages, there is a continuing process of interiorization, that life psychologically contracts. The positive aspect of this turn of attention inward is that it enables an inner exploration that may help us find a meaning and wholeness in life that makes it possible to accept death. In Jung, we see the abstract beginnings of a theory of normal psychological aging that, along with the work of Buhler, stresses age-appropriate coping behaviors and tasks. With the work of Erikson, we see a slightly more specific approach to the tasks of old age.

Erikson: The Resolutions of Psychosocial Tasks

Like Buhler and Jung, Erik Erikson also saw the need to understand the process of personality development throughout the life cycle. Somewhat more specifically, however, Erikson delineated eight stages of development, each representing a psychosocial crisis or task defined by a combination of cultural and maturational needs. The successful resolution of each of these stage-related crises is thought to determine our self-evaluation, our success in adapting to both inner psychic and socially imposed tasks, and the future development of personality. A brief summary of Erikson's eight stages, psychosocial crises, and the psychological quality derived from successful resolution of each crisis is given in Table 3–1.

Although Erikson has stipulated that each of the eight crises is not necessarily bound to a specific age, he does maintain that there is a strong likelihood that each crisis is in the foreground at the appropriate stage. He also notes that individuals probably oscillate between two stages at any point in the life cycle and the resolution of earlier crises affects successful entry into later stages.[11] Table 3–1 shows that the psychosocial crisis most prevalent in old age is integrity versus despair.

Such a conflict involves the task of reconciling to one's satisfaction that one's life has had purpose and meaning. It involves ". . . the acceptance of one's own and only life cycle and of the people who have become significant to it as something that had to be and that, by necessity, permitted no substitution.[12] The opposite side of the coin is *despair*, the feeling that time is too short for making radical changes in life or that alternate roads are no longer possible. Erikson tells us:

> . . . this is why the elderly try to "doctor" their memories. Rationalized bitterness and disgust can mask that despair, which in severe psychopathology aggravates a senile syndrome of depression, hypochondria, and paranoiac hate. For, whatever chance to transcend the limitations of his self seems to depend on his full (if often tragic) engagement in the one and only life cycle permitted to him.[13]

Erikson goes on to remind us that the task faced by older people is not the total victory of integrity *over* despair and disgust, but rather, the achievement of a favorable balance in integrity's favor. According to his formulation, both experiences are inevitable in old age. The experience of despair is there for all old people, no matter how much they have achieved or how much they take on a realistic

TABLE 3–1. ERIKSON'S STAGES, PSYCHOSOCIAL CRISES, AND OUTCOMES OF SUCCESSFUL RESOLUTIONS

Stage	Psychosocial Crises	Outcome (if resolved)
Infancy	Trust versus mistrust	Hope
Early childhood	Autonomy versus shame, doubt	Will
Play age	Initiative versus guilt	Purpose
School age	Industry versus inferiority	Competence
Adolescence	Identity versus identity confusion	Fidelity
Young adulthood	Intimacy versus isolation	Love
Maturity	Generativity versus self-absorption	Care
Old age	Integrity versus despair, disgust	Wisdom

Adapted from Erikson, E. H. Reflections on Dr. Borg's life cycle. Daedalus, *1976,* 105, 22.

attitude about life. Erikson's theory, then, implies that those working with the aged should not necessarily encourage the denial of death, but rather, the assimilation of its reality into the experience of life, just as integrity should absorb and assimilate the inevitable experiences of despair.

The appropriate resolution of the conflict of integrity versus despair, therefore, results in a sense of wisdom, which is "the detached and yet active concern with life itself in the face of death itself, and that it maintains and conveys the integrity of experience, in spite of the decline of bodily and mental functions."[14]

Peck: Expansion of Erikson's Theory

Although Erikson, Buhler, and Jung addressed issues of personality development in later life, their observations and descriptions might be considered rather global and generalized. In this light, Peck attempted to further delineate and specify the issues that are crucial in old age.[15] He also specified what he thought were the crucial issues of middle age as they relate to issues in later life (Table 3–2).

TABLE 3–2. DESCRIPTION AND OUTLINE OF PECK'S STAGES AND PSYCHOLOGICAL ISSUES OF LATER LIFE

Stage	Psychological Issue	Description
Middle age	1. Valuing wisdom versus valuing physical powers	Successful aging involves the ability to rely on life experience and cognitive abilities, rather than physical strength or stamina. Depression can result if the shift is not made.
	2. Socializing versus sexualizing in human relationships	Aging persons must reconcile the appearance of the sexual climacteric by allowing the sexual element in their relationships to play a lessened role. New and deeper emphasis on friendship and companionship aspects can potentially improve and strengthen marital and other interpersonal relations.
	3. Cathectic flexibility versus cathective impoverishment	Cathectic (or emotional) flexibility is the capacity to make new relationships in the face of inevitable losses as children leave home, parents die, and friendship patterns change. It is crucial for successful aging. Positive adaptation to aging requires the development of a *generalized* set of behaviors to making new as well as redefining existing emotional relationships (as when children grow up).

TABLE 3–2. (Cont.)

Stage	Psychological Issue	Description
	4. Mental flexibility versus mental rigidity	The ability to remain open to new ideas and to learn from new experiences, as opposed to being dominated by a set of inflexible rules "automatically" governing behavior, is important for a continuing sense of growth in later life.
Old age	1. Ego differentiation versus work–role preoccupation	Successful adaptation to old age may require the establishment of a variety of valued activities and new roles to modify the impact of occupational loss or change in parental and other roles.
	2. Body transcendence versus body preoccupation	The ability to focus on the comforts and enjoyments of social interactions and mental tasks while deemphasizing body pains and frailties.
	3. Ego transcendence versus ego preoccupation	Stresses the importance of living as unselfishly and generously as possible in order to ensure that one's personal death is not as important in comparison to the awareness that through children, through contributions to the culture, or through one's friendships, one's actions will remain significant beyond one's lifetime. Though death is inevitable, human beings can experience a sense of gratification and meaning about their lives in the future potential of their ideas, family, or future generations of the species.

Adapted from Peck, R. C. Psychological developments in the second half of life. In J. E. Anderson (Ed.), Psychological aspects of aging. *Washington D.C.: American Psychological Association, 1956, pp. 44–49.*

Peck describes middle age as being on a continuum that leads to old age. By comparing polar extremes, he offers a model of what may be conceptualized as successful aging compared to nonsuccessful aging, similar to Erikson's view.

Butler: The Life Review Process

What can be considered successful adjustment during old age? What personality characteristic facilitates the acceptance of later life stages? One phenomenon that many people associate specifically with old age is reminiscence. Although lay people may attribute this concern for past events shown by older individuals as escape from the present or as senility, reminiscence has been found to serve a number of useful functions in the psychological organization of the aged. For example, Butler, a research psychiatrist, has theorized that reminiscence is part of a normal and healthy *life review process* brought about by the realization of the closeness of death.[16] Manifestations of the life review include mirror-gazing, nostalgia, interests in storytelling, reconsideration of past activities, and flashes of extreme clarity about early life events. During the life review, it is not uncommon for some older people to "spill out" their life story to anyone who will listen, while other older people may speak in a monologue without apparent concern for the presence or absence of others.[17] Those who work with the aged must train themselves to listen thoughtfully instead of ignoring such reminiscences, for they may serve a therapeutic function.

It should be stressed that the life review will probably lead to some negative feelings and regrets. In its more severe forms, it can lead to feelings of depression, anxiety, guilt, despair, and obsessional ruminations about past mistakes. On balance, however, the life review can, for many people (especially if they had been fairly well integrated in earlier life), yield positive results, such as healing old disputes with enemies, attempting to right old wrongs, correcting any changes in negative attitudes toward relatives or friends, engendering a sense of pride in one's achievements, and culminating in a feeling of personal serenity—perhaps related to the belief that one has done his or her best in life. Such creative works as memoirs, scrapbooks, family albums, and other interests kindled in old age also may be results of the life review. For these latter reasons, the sensitive worker should encourage this process if it appears beneficial.

Interpreting the Life Review

Two ways of interpreting the life review process are suggested.[18] One is based on Erikson's model, which thinks of the life review as "the fulfillment of the life task of the last phase of life." In this model, the life review is a means of warding off despair and permitting the older person to accept the ending of life with good feeling. Another point of view focuses on the model conceived by Alfred Adler.[19] This approach says that the life review is effective because one has come to recognize that life is a "series of crises and protracted struggles and that he has persevered in the past and triumphed." Viewed this way, the client looks ahead to the new demands of life with the same optimism that helped him or her to master those of the past. This approach emphasizes enthusiastically the positives in the person's life. If it does not, the author suggests that "the life review can become counterproductive and convince the patient that life has been one failure after another." The therapist is advised to first consider whether the client's past, racked up in the life review process, is a "firm foundation for present coping, or an impediment." Initial interviews with the prospective life-review client should provide answers. If he or she has successfully met problems throughout life, a life review is suggested; when an entire life has been viewed as a failure, a life review is not advised.

SUMMARY OF STAGE-THEORISTS' VIEW

Stage theorists see development as the successful completion of new tasks. They place little emphasis, however, on what the quality of life is like in old age. The exception to this is Robert Butler, who makes the following succinct points:

1. Older people are involved with the present. While they may reflect upon the past in an attempt to integrate it into present experience, it is the experience of the present that is important.
2. The older adult has accumulated wisdom and experience. This wealth of life's resources can then be offered to younger people. The older adult can be an excellent resource person, counselor, or advisor.
3. Older people wish to pass on power. As such, they are attached to those objects that are important to them. Old possessions are valued. Part of this valuing is an attempt to hand them on to future generations, possibly as a way of ensuring immortality.[20]

EXAMINING DEATH AS PART OF LIFE

While stage theorists divide life into stages, others are involved with the process of life and its inevitable consequence—death. The theme of man's immortality, as we have seen, dominates much of the thinking in the gerontological literature. Focusing on the theme of death is one way to explore more fully the force called "life."

The Death Process: Death Anxiety

As in Samuel Beckett's play, "Waiting for Godot," in which the main characters wait and wait, a common assumption that we make about older people is that they sit, aimless and anxious, waiting to die. As with so many of our myths about aging, this is untrue. Most older people are well, live in the community and, as "survivors," are made up of the sterner stuff that makes for living a longer life. They are involved in life, not death. A test of subjects from 30 to 80 years of age, assessing "death anxiety," found no relationship between age and any degree of death anxiety.[21] This was in accord with other findings.[22] One study, involving 2,500 people aged 19 to 85, from a variety of populations (including psychiatric patients, adolescents, and parents of adolescents), reflected no relationship between age and fear of death. Apparently, despite our beliefs that the elderly do nothing but contemplate death, scientific research has shown that age *per se* is *not* a crucial determinant of the level of death anxiety or preoccupation with death. Personality factors and life experiences are the key determinants in fearing death. Curiously, one finding reports high levels of death anxiety, along with general anxiety and depression, in senior high school students. This group is compared with junior high school students and evening college students. The authors focus on the high stress levels experienced by these adolescent students as they deal with new stages of emotional and physical growth.[23] Conversely, it may be that the elderly, having faced all of life, can now face death realistically and without undue denial, anxiety, or fear of the inevitable.

Kubler-Ross: Personality Organization and the Process of Dying

It is only in recent history that specific attempts have been made to understand whether there are psychologically "normal" styles of responding to the harsh reality of death. One of the more sensitive attempts to understand personality changes in the terminally ill was carried out by Kubler-Ross, a psychiatrist and researcher who interviewed a large number of dying patients and who has developed a stage theory of the dying process.[24] Kubler-Ross's theory proposes that the process of dying normally consists of an orderly progression of five adaptive stages. Although she assumes that these stages follow one another in a sequential order, others have noted that the terminally ill may oscillate among all or some of the stages as often as every few hours.[25] We therefore believe that it is more helpful to consider the following five stages as distinguishable, but not necessarily sequential, crisis periods in the dying process.[26]

Denial and Isolation. The initial response to the awareness of death may be a temporary state of shock and numbness, followed by the feeling that it "must be a mistake." The vast majority of patients interviewed by Kubler-Ross held onto their need for denial for relatively short periods; only 3 of 200 interviewed held onto this denial to the very last.

This initial defensive process is seen as beneficial because it gives the patient time to develop less-stringent defenses to cope with the reality of the situation. This initial denial should be respected as a normal and healthy process of coping with unpleasant and shocking news. Nurses and others who work with the terminally ill should not attempt to prematurely discuss a patient's feelings. The patient will reveal a willingness to deal with the issue of death when he or she acknowledges the reality of the situation.

Although premature discouragement of denial is not useful, Kubler-Ross also notes that hospital workers who, for their own reasons, feel the need to deny the patient's impending death may encourage the ill to maintain a pretense of well-being. Kubler-Ross adds that the sensitive worker should expect terminal patients who have gone beyond the denial stage to occasionally and, throughout their illness, momentarily isolate this reality from their awareness.

Anger. As the patient's denial of impending death diminishes, a new feeling of anger, envy, and resentment, best summarized as "why me?", emerges. No one is exempt from this anger, for the patient seems to be struggling to blame somebody for this overwhelming disaster. Often hospital personnel, relatives, and friends may become targets. Kubler-Ross advises that it is crucial for those who work with or visit the dying to recognize the symptoms of the *anger stage* and not take such behavior personally. She observes that a staff or family member who reacts personally may tend to curtail visits and otherwise avoid the patient who, in reality, needs their attention and care. Anger must be recognized as the beginning of an acceptance of the reality of one's death.

Bargaining. Once the anger subsides, many terminally ill patients engage in forms of bargaining patterns. It is as if he or she is trying to make a deal with fate by changing the strategy from one of anger to asking for a favor. Kubler-Ross sees this behavior as similar to the maneuver of the child who, denied permission to visit a friend overnight, turns the anger into the query, "If I am very good all week and wash the dishes every evening, then will you let me go?" In this way, many terminally ill patients attempt to gain postponements, often by making secret deals with God. Kubler-Ross suggests that some bargains may be expressions of long-standing, unresolved guilt, such as offerings to be righteous or to do church work, and might be resolved usefully by staff, if so recognized.

Depression. Eventually, the terminally ill patient becomes depressed. (This experience may be precipitated by the need for further surgery, more symptoms, or physical changes caused by the illness.) Denial, anger, and bargaining become replaced with a sense of great loss. Kubler-Ross notes that two kinds of depression may be observed: a reactive depression and a preparatory depression. *Reactive depression* is the sense of shame and sadness that results from the removal of valued physical features (such as that experienced by a woman whose uterus or breast was removed because of cancer). *Preparatory depression* involves a sense of sadness precipitated by the realization of impending losses through one's own death. Both forms of depression should be identified and dealt with in different ways.

Reactive depression may be dealt with by directly attempting to enhance the patient's self-esteem, such as providing a prosthesis for the breast-cancer victim or complimenting a woman for some especially feminine feature if she no longer feels "like a woman" because of her surgery. In these situations, good cheer and frequent visiting may be of some help.

Preparatory depression should not, according to Kubler-Ross, be dealt with by direct attempts to cheer up the patient. Encouragements and reassurances are not as helpful for patients in this phase. Instead, Kubler-Ross suggests that the patient be allowed to fully express his or her sorrow. Often, sitting silently and quietly interacting by touching or holding the person's hand (just "being with" the person) may be enough to help the patient gain a personal acceptance of impending death.

Acceptance. If death has not been sudden or unexpected, and if there has been time to work through the first four stages, the patient will reach the point of acceptance. During this final stage, the terminally ill person seems "almost void of feelings." Tired and weak, he or she senses that the "struggle" is over and that the time for the final rest before the long journey has come. It is during this stage that the family may need more attention and support than does the dying person. In part, the family may not understand that the patient may wish to be left alone much of the time or does not feel talkative with even the closest family members. Again, as in the preparatory-depression phase, quiet, emphathic communication, such as holding the patient's hand, is all that is really desired.

In discussing the foregoing five stages of the normal ways of coping with death, Kubler-Ross elucidates some important guidelines for those who work with the terminally ill and the aged. She clearly demystifies the last stage of one's life for family members and friends of dying patients. Her general sensitivity to the topic leads her to one final insight—the notion that the phenomenon of *hope* is underneath it all, stabilizing the dying person's ability to live through the weeks and months of suffering. She also suggests that staff, by reinforcing this idea, can aid in this normal and healthy process.

The general sensitivity of Kubler-Ross to the topic is remarkable, and her outline of what attitudes to recognize is as humanistic as it is practical. We must, however, insert a note of caution about her view and its implications for practical use.[27] Researchers have noted that her theory is not yet a proven fact or empirically demonstrated but, rather, that it stands as a significant clinical report on the personal experiences of dying patients by essentially one observer. A second criticism of her theory is that it does not take into account potential differences between males and females. For example, it appears that women may be more upset by the impact of their death on others, while males may feel more concerned with their loss of stature or power. It also has been pointed out that the nature of the disease, the ethnic identity of the patient, his or her life-long personality or cognitive style, and the immediate environment (an alienating nursing home or the same house in which the person was born) must be taken into account.

Those who work with the aged, however, should be careful to distinguish between what usually happens and what theory says *should* happen during the dying process. Kubler-Ross herself cautioned that dying patients should not be rushed through the various stages. As with any theory, the Kubler-Ross stages should be viewed as useful guidelines through which we may gain an increased understanding of the normal psychological changes to be expected in the last phase of life.

THE CULTURAL CONTEXT OF THE AGING PROCESS

Previously, we discussed the biological processes and aspects of normal personality development in old age. In order to more fully understand the complex of forces that influence who the aged are, we must focus on the cultural context in which the aged live. What does society expect old people to be like? What are these expectations based on, and what implications do these expectations have for the problems encountered by those who work with the aged?

Cultural Definitions

The criteria used to define old age vary from society to society. In many simple cultures, old age is defined in functional terms—the point at which biological deterioration literally prevents the individual from carrying out his or her traditional work or other valuable role functions. In these societies, the old are the "about to die," not those who have reached some particular chronological age. This definition of old age is very different from the formal chronological criterion that typifies American society.[28] In this society, old age begins at age 65. Many people do not

seem to realize that this criterion is purely cultural and is a definition originally based on the traditional start of eligibility for Social Security benefits.

We might suspect that, as the retirement age changes, the cultural definitions of when old age begins will also change. Early retirement, however (whether brought about by affluence or planned unemployment), may pose new problems for those who need to discover meaningful substitute activities. The importance of this issue is heightened by recent estimates that indicate that the average member of society will soon spend more than half of his or her life outside the labor force.[29] Indeed, the setting of progressively earlier retirement ages, in combination with the phenomenon of increasing longevity, will probably cause a series of socially induced psychological problems; our society may be creating a new life stage that contains no specific role definitions for the aged. The problem is further compounded by the cultural tendency of Americans to downgrade nonwork or leisure activities upon retirement.[30]

Roles and Norms

The concept of social role is an important one for understanding the position of the aged in our society. For present purposes, a *role* may be defined as a content area within a social system that has specific action characteristics. For example, the roles of mother, father, truck driver, student, and spouse are reasonably identifiable content areas within our American social system that carry with them specific kinds of behaviors (or action characteristics) that are readily predictable. Most people, if asked to play-act a "student" or "truck driver," could do so without having to know much about individual personality characteristics. All students study or read or sit in classes, for example. That certain roles are predictable and that the behaviors they imply are very specific can also be seen by the fact that we can quickly identify someone who performs outside an appropriate role—for example, the 75-year-old woman who wears a bikini or the 80-year-old man who develops an interest in sky diving.

These examples may be construed to indicate that certain roles are probably considered inappropriate for an elderly person in terms of current social norms. It is not considered "right" to show off one's body or engage in dangerous sports unless one is young or has a certain physical build. Role behaviors, then, are governed by normative prescriptions—what we should be doing as fathers, mothers, men, women, or students. The development, acceptance, and internalization of these "shoulds" may be called the process of socialization. It is through this process, which involves exposure to parents, the educational system, the mass media, peer pressures, and more, that one learns to perform particular roles in terms of the social norms of any given society. It is only when a society does not socialize individuals for appropriate roles or has not as yet defined the appropriate roles (as may be the case for long periods of retirement and old age in the United States) that problems in adjustment may ensue.

We should also be aware that societies vary greatly in terms of the roles and norms for which they socialize their participants. When an individual learns one set of norms and roles but then emigrates to a new and different society, he or she may

have great difficulty in adjusting and may be considered deviant or even mentally ill. Psychiatrists and psychologists sometimes encounter problems in diagnosing the adjustment of foreign-born or recently arrived elderly who believe in spiritualism. To those aged, hearing and seeing spirits, and experiencing visitations, may be very normal and are related to roles learned in their previous cultural settings. It is important that those who work with the aged are aware of the possibility that behavior in the elderly that may appear bizarre or deviant by this society's current norms may be the product of the anticipation of aging in another culture or may be the results of values learned in another time period.

Age Grading and Anticipatory Socialization

Age grading refers to the notion that all societies organize the life span into stages or time periods, during which an individual is expected to do certain things (attend school, marry, work, retire, and even to die) or to behave in certain ways (play in childhood, be achievement-oriented in youth, and be nonsexual in old age). Age grades are chronological aspects of social norms.

There have been some indications that age grading can pose a great problem for the aged in our society. In a study of mentally well and mentally ill elderly, Clark found that the value orientations considered healthy for younger and middle-aged people were often associated with mental illness in old age.[31] She noted that those elderly diagnosed as mentally ill seemed to cling to precisely those patterns of value orientation upheld as most representative of the core values and norms of American society in the years when they had been middle-aged persons—the values and norms of individualism, competitiveness, aggressiveness, acquisitiveness of money, and future orientation. Clark implies that mental illness in old age may involve an inability to give up previously held values and move into the next age grade. She concludes that normal aging in our society depends on the acceptance of a culturally prescribed value shift (or age grade) imposed upon those entering old-age status.

Age grading may also serve useful purposes, especially if we think of its role in the process of anticipatory socialization. *Anticipatory socialization* is the process of preparing for a change in role or status. It involves the ability—and time—to explore and try out new norms or expectations that will be associated with a new role or status once the change is made.

Simple societies, for example, tend to provide ample opportunity for anticipatory socialization. Close interaction with the elders in the small populations of these societies provides an opportunity to model, identify, and become familiar with the roles and norms characteristic of the aged. Since, in such societies, average longevity is low, the ratio of elders to the available "job slots" and ceremonial positions is also low. Because of these factors, the middle-aged in simple societies often have "something" they can actually look forward to doing, or being, when they reach old age. Many anthropological studies have thus found a positive correlation between the existence of age grades and the continuation into important political, religious, or ceremonial offices of aged men.[32]

Unlike many tribal societies, in which the young member knows that he will

inevitably accede to the status of leader—if he survives—American society does not seem to provide a set of clearly defined role expectations and norms for the elderly. If we note that American society has more people who live longer proportionately than do most tribal groups (because of such factors as improved child care), we can see that complete anticipatory socialization may be, at least, a difficult task for the young and middle-aged generations. The task of discovering new roles for old age is further complicated by the high value placed on individual development and freedom of action in the United States.

Some social scientists have noted that, at least for the urban, affluent aged, a new set of norms involving the general value of activity (as opposed to work) is becoming institutionalized.[33] Upon retirement, leisure, "as long as it is marked by some activity, has become a value in American life."[34] It seems that, as long as Americans are "doing something" or "keeping busy," they may feel useful and worthwhile. The trend toward age-segregated retirement communities in which affluent elderly pursue active lives, independent of their children, may become a new norm for which anticipatory socialization is to be inaugurated. The cost of such a norm may be very high, in the sense that it perpetuates the physical and psychological separation of the older and younger generations and may, in the long run, be very detrimental to the future of our social organization. Further, such a norm does not solve the problems encountered by the poor or economically deprived elderly, who make up a substantial proportion of our population.

Although age grading may be beneficial, because it helps the elderly through the process of anticipatory socialization to become familiar with and accept their new status, the American version may be ultimately dysfunctional, in that anticipatory socialization involves age segregation that encourages separateness between the generations. These factors must be kept in mind by all those who work with the aged.

Attitudes Toward Aging

A major impact of the socialization process in any society involves its effect on the formation of attitudes toward aging and the aged. If American society most clearly emphasizes the value of norms and roles relevant to work and achievement orientation, so that people are valued for their utility instead of their worth, we might expect that most people would not look forward to growing old. The kinds of feelings toward aging that are engendered by society also may have critical effects on the capacity of people to adjust—or even survive—in old age. Bennett and Eckman noted that those elderly who have negative attitudes toward their own aging may lack the motivation to seek needed services, health care, or other assistance. In addition, older people's negative attitudes toward aging may alienate younger members of the community and may increase the gap between age groups.[35] Positive attitudes, however, might engender understanding and empathy for a life stage that most Americans will live to experience. In this light, we turn to a brief survey of research on attitudes toward aging among various age groups, including the aged themselves.

Problems in Research on Attitudes Toward the Elderly

While research on attitudes toward the elderly was initiated over 30 years ago,[36] results have often been conflicting. Though many studies report negativism toward the aged, by young and old alike, research methods have been cited as being inadequate.[37] Some of the problems plaguing gerontologists have been cited as: the lack of a formal attitude-assessment instrument; the kinds of instructions given to participants, young and old alike; the lack of distinction between items in a questionnaire that are clearly attitudinal: "They (old people) have too much power in business and politics" and those actual beliefs, such as, "They do not participate in sports.[38]" Yet, despite these problems, we present some of the most instrumental attitudes toward aging.

Some Pioneer Studies on Attitudes Toward Aging

Among the first to study attitudes toward aging were Tuckman and Lorge. They developed a simple questionnaire that presumably tapped negative stereotypes and misconceptions about various aspects of aging. Their questionnaire consisted of statements about old people (to which respondents answered either yes or no), such as: "Old people need glasses to read." "They are in the happiest period of their lives." "They get upset easily." "They just like to sit and dream."[39]

In general, study of the Tuckman and Lorge questionnaire supports the view that old people are devalued by both young and old respondents. One interesting study, which used a modified version of the Tuckman–Lorge questionnaire, was conducted by Axelrod and Eisdorfer. They asked a sample of college students to give their opinions on the Tuckman–Lorge items as they related to five age categories: 35, 45, 55, 65, and 75. The results showed that the ascription of negative attitudes by the young people increased for each decade from 35 to 75 years.[40]

A slightly different approach used to tap attitudes toward old people consists of sentence-completion tests.[41] This method involves the presentation of short sentence stems, such as: "In general, old people need . . ." which respondents then complete as they wish. Research using the sentence-completion format shows that the young and the old differ in their attitudes and beliefs about old age and old people. Here are some examples of the ways in which different age groups have responded to sentence completion.

One of the Greatest Fears of Many Old People Is. . . . Younger respondents tended to consider "death or dying" as the greatest fear. Older people stressed "lack of money" and "financial insecurity." In analyzing this response, the authors suggest that closeness to death may not necessarily imply an increased fear of death at the conscious level. They speculate that a denial process may be at work among the older respondents. They also note that the differences between old and young respondents on this question point out the existence of cross-generational differences in understanding the problems of the aged.

Old People Tend to Resent. . . . Kogan and Shelton found that the young respondents tended to cite themselves or the general category of "younger people" as the object of old people's resentments. Older respondents were more specific in their answers, referring to "rejection," "lack of concern," and "reference to age." The authors suggest that the old people were somewhat concerned (at least implicitly) with the attitudes of the young toward them.

In 1977, Palmore developed a Facts on Aging quiz, a widely accepted true–false test reflecting an individual's knowledge of 25 facts on aging. Some of the results showed the existence of very widespread misconceptions about the aged, including how many old persons there are in the population, how many are in institutions, the degree of poverty among them, and so on. Similarly, in 1975, the Harris Poll, interviewing over 4,000 people 18 years old and over, showed that most of those interviewed associated aging with passive activities. Most people over 65, they stated, watched TV, sat and thought, or slept. Again, in an extensive 1973 survey, Bennett and Eckman reported that "negative views of aging are shared by young and old alike."[42] That attitudes about age are related to self-esteem was found in a study conducted by Ward (1977). He interviewed community-living older persons (over age 60) and found that attitude toward aging was a good predictor of self-esteem.

Attitudes continue to be researched. In a more recent survey, it was found that, when people aged 18 to 59 are asked to make judgments of old and young persons alike, negativism toward old age is expressed.[43] When these same people are asked to make judgments only of old people, there is little evidence of aging stereotypes! In this study, females were less negative than males, as were those with nonminority ethnic status, though caution is suggested in interpreting these results.

While attitudes toward the elderly continue to be researched, findings are often less than conclusive. In a 1985 study, the authors suggest that, during the past 30 to 40 years, society has tended to view older people in a more positive light and to see them as "contributors," while other groups (including the alcoholic, drug addict, and ex-convict) are seen mostly negatively.[44] This study identifies as a "social myth" perpetuated by the gerontological literature the idea that attitudes toward the aged are pervasively negative. Yet, for the most part, attitudes toward the elderly are still revealed as less than positive.

That mental-health practitioners are affected by these attitudes is obvious, for all of us are part of this society. This was demonstrated in research showing that health-care providers working with the elderly *preferred* to work with patients who had "disease-related symptoms" rather than with clients with "normal aging" problems.[45] It's no wonder that the older adult responds to these attitudes with behaviors sometimes interpreted as defensive or super-cautious.

The Culture of Caution

In summarizing their research, we noted that Kogan and Shelton imply that older people may be somewhat defensive about how others see them, that they probably try to anticipate the feelings of the younger generation in order to gain acceptance, and that they try to avoid the possibility of rejection by that dominant majority. Indeed, this socially induced defensiveness may be the cause of the high degree of cautiousness shown among the aged, a cautiousness that may have been erroneously interpreted as evidence that the old lack the ability to do certain tasks.

The belief that older people are more conservative in their approach to life than are their younger counterparts, and that there is a generation gap of caution, seems to have been accepted by social scientists for many decades. In fact, the popular belief that the aged are uncomfortable with the new and the uncertain, expect failure, fear rejection, have a low degree of self-confidence, and avoid obtaining information about their abilities has been documented by the research literature.[46] We shall now look at some of the research evidence and at the possibility that cultural factors might explain much of the need for certainty and low risk-taking evidenced by the aged.

Errors of Omission. As a group, the aged are more likely to commit errors of omission instead of errors of commission. An error of omission involves a nonresponse (such as not answering a question on a test). An error of commission involves making a mistake (for example, providing the wrong answer on a test or making a wrong decision instead of not deciding). The omission error may stem from a desire for certainty or as a way of avoiding failure and increasing self-esteem. The virtue of this approach is that older people tend to make few mistakes on tasks if given enough time.[47] Many of the elderly, therefore, do not do well on intelligence tests because these often require answers within specific time limits.

Risk Taking. The tendency toward caution among the aged seems to exist, not only where abilities or capacities are at issue, but also where choices, preferences, or certain behaviors are called for. Wallach and Kogan found that older people were considerably more cautious than the young (especially when making decisions on financial matters) on a risk-taking questionnaire.[48] This consisted of 12 "everyday-life situations" involving dilemmas of choice. Each situation described a central person who is supposed to choose between two courses of action. One course in each situation was very risky but involved the possibility of considerable gain if successful. Each young or old respondent was faced with the task of "advising" the person in each of the 12 situations on what degree of certainty he or she should require before choosing the risky alternative.

The choices ranged from 10 percent certainty (great risk) to 90 percent certainty (low risk). Respondents also had the option of choosing the most conservative alternative; that is, of making *no* decision to follow the risky course of action. An example of one such choice dilemma follows:

> Mr. A., an electrical engineer who is married and has one child, has been working for a large electronics corporation since graduating from college five years ago. He is assured of a lifetime job with a modest, though adequate, salary and liberal pension benefits upon retirement. On the other hand, it is very unlikely that his salary will increase much before he retires. While attending a convention, Mr. A. is offered a job with a small, newly founded company with a highly uncertain future. The new job would pay more to start and would offer the possibility of a share in the ownership if the company survived the competition of the larger firms.[49]

Respondents were asked whether they would consider it worthwhile to "advise" Mr. A. to take the new job (or would advise that no decision be made).

The Wallach–Kogan findings have been criticized for not being totally relevant to the aged and have since been modified by Botwinick.[50] Botwinick also found that the elderly were more cautious in their approach to risky decisions than were the younger people.

Although the elderly may indeed appear more cautious, this is not the complete story, especially for those who intend to work with the aged. The original Wallach–Kogan items allowed the respondent to choose a no-risk alternative; to advise not taking the new job in the case of Mr. A. Botwinick's items also contained this option. Further analysis of his results showed that the elderly have a very strong tendency to choose this no-risk alternative. What does this mean in terms of decision-making processes in the aged? What happens when older subjects are not given the option of choosing a no-risk alternative? Although we might logically expect that they would then opt for the next most conservative choices available (i.e., 90 percent certainty), this is, in fact, not the case. When a new questionnaire compelled both young and old respondents to take *some* degree of risk, age differences in cautiousness were not seen at all.[51]

Thus, when risk cannot be avoided, older people may be as venturesome as their younger counterparts. The only time that they seem to be cautious (at least in experimental settings) is when this caution is a permissible alternative. Older people may not really be reluctant to be somewhat risky (or venturesome) if the situation demands it. What seems to be required is that the situation be specifically structured to enable the elderly to function in this capacity. Many real-life situations, however, do not involve clearly structured demands or activities. One exception is certain aspects of the world of work and, as we have seen, the aged are virtually excluded from this world through Social Security and automatic retirement laws. This leaves only the area of leisure for many of the aged. Leisure, however, is unstructured time, a domain of experience in which we have the opportunity to exercise maximal choice, and leisure settings may not afford the demands to be venturesome that some older people might need.[52]

Brok and Westcott studied the free-time preferences of people in adolescence, young adulthood, adulthood, and old age.[53] When asked to choose, from a list of options, how they preferred to spend their free time, older people wanted activities involving a great deal of order and preplanning. This was the opposite of younger respondents, who least preferred such activities. The younger and adult groups most wanted activities involving social affiliation and private autonomy needs. The high preference shown for "order" by the older people in this study might be indicative of the tendency, given the option, for the aged to feel more comfortable about time that they can structure and control—perhaps, in a way, analogous to the low-risk findings discussed earlier.

But if the elderly are really not that cautious in situations that prevent them from exercising the cautious option, we still need to explain why they choose the certain, more conservative road whenever possible. One explanation favored by the present authors involves the values and socialization effects of American society. Our culture is oriented toward the young, and there seem to be few healthy norms available to the old. One of the few norms in existence may be reflected by the attitude and risk studies just cited. Indeed, perhaps there is a norm of caution, socially induced and culturally backed, to which society expects the elderly person to adhere almost magically upon retirement.

The probability that such traits are socially influenced rather than strictly biological arises from the fact that, if called upon, the aged do show the same risk-taking tendencies as the young. This is not to say that there are no real changes with age. It seems, instead, that the elderly act as they are expected to but are devalued by the young, who live by a different set of values. We then have a self-fulfilling prophecy: What is expected of the old is confirmed when they conform, and their conformity is then devalued.

Could it be that "there may well be a conspiracy on the part of the middle-aged to remove the old from active participation in society"?[54] Some deficits observed in intelligence tests given to the aged may be the results of socially induced policies. As Schaie notes:

> . . . at least some older people do less well when they are afraid of involvement in a task involving unreasonable risk of loss or embarrassment, but that careful control of instructional set may well induce the older person to consider alternatives he might otherwise eschew.[55]

Schaie suggests that one solution to the dilemma of the old is for workers in the field to use the knowledge that the aged will show a normal predilection toward risk taking if given no choice. Compulsory-education requirements might be set up for older populations (as they are for younger) or, alternatively, adequate reinforcements or reward contingencies could be made available for voluntary participation in educational programs. These suggestions imply that structured or "moderately challenging" incentives might be a way to motivate many of the aged in order to counteract the detrimental effects of culturally induced cautiousness.

THE ENVIRONMENT OF THE AGED

All human behavior is influenced by the environmental context in which it occurs, as well as by individual biological and psychological factors. It is only through comprehension of, first, the physical, social, and interpersonal influences that exist "outside" the person and, second, the interaction of these influences with the unique characteristics of any particular person that we can begin to understand human behavior. We also know that, as people age, environmental factors seem to play a role of increasing importance in their behavior. In part, the stronger influence of environmental factors among the elderly results from, not only their lowered ability to cope with socially induced stress, but also from decreases in their physiological competence.[56] It seems clear that those who work with the aged must learn to pay particular attention to the impact of environmental factors.

Living Arrangements

In general, living arrangements of the elderly vary from residential single-family houses to highly institutionalized nursing homes. Between these two extremes, there are a number of other options for living that are increasing in use. Many older people reside in mobile home parks, which are less expensive than houses but which retain some measure of privacy and a sense of independence. Others, especially in the middle- and upper-income groups, turn to retirement villages. In urban areas, housing projects and retirement hotels, often of varying quality, are important residential sites.

It is a misconception that most of the elderly live in some form of institution. Recent studies show that 70 percent of individuals over age 65 actually own their own homes.[57] Unfortunately, those who are homeowners are not exempt from the considerable economic stresses faced by all elderly, who (on average) fall among the lowest income groups in the United States. Repair costs, utility bills, and high property taxes may become major environmental stressors that, in turn, may cause maladaptive coping patterns. Some of the elderly, for example, attempt to compromise by purchasing less (or lower-quality) food in order to maintain their homes or apartments. Many are forced to move to, or remain in, substandard housing, which (in turn) creates a spiral of despair and withdrawal. It has been suggested that economic stresses in general can lead to a lowered sense of self-esteem and depression in some of the aged.[58]

Age Segregation

Whether it is better for older people to live in an environment that separates them from other age groups instead of living in age-integrated settings remains unclear. Age-integrated settings, which provide physical proximity between young and old, do not necessarily guarantee that the two age groups will relate socially. The evidence that cross-generational friendships are encouraged by having different age groups live in close proximity is very weak.[59] In comparison, age-segregated living arrangements, particularly in secure and well-managed apartment buildings or projects, appear to encourage social interaction among elderly tenants, especially among those who live on the same floor.[60]

Although age segregation may be beneficial because it encourages interaction and provides a degree of peer security among the elderly, it may be philosophically negative to perpetuate such living arrangements. The continued separation of age groups in our society may only increase and reinforce the overwhelmingly negative stereotypes and lack of knowledge that the young have about old age. One solution might be to establish multi-aged community centers in areas of age-segregated housing. Such centers might serve as common meeting grounds through which the old and the young could interact while not necessarily living in the same housing.

Mobility and the Everyday Environment

A brief stroll through most urban and suburban areas in the United States quickly leads to the realization that the physical environment is designed for the active adult, not for small children or the handicapped, and especially not for the aged. It is as if the elderly had been ''vetoed out'' of society by architects and designers.[61] Environmental design features such as steep steps to subway or commuter trains, inadequately lit street signs, traffic lights that change rapidly (thereby failing to give some older people sufficient time to cross the street), and insufficient or expensive public transportation are all factors that can affect the mobility and exploratory desires of older people. One study found that the New York urban elderly rarely left their immediate neighborhood and that they lived within a constricted social space.[62]

Prosthetic Environments

A prosthetic device is an artificial part, such as a limb, which may help one to function. As applied to environments, the idea of a prosthesis suggests that the aged may be helped to function by the use of proper design features. The concept of a prosthetic environment for the elderly has been discussed in terms of the following categories:

1. *Life-maintenance activity*. This stresses the importance of physical safety, such as nonskid floors in a house.
2. *Perceptual behavior*. Lawton notes that the use of bright colors can enhance orientation to place as well as overcome the depressive ''aesthetic barrenness'' of some institutional environments. Poor eyesight, suffered by many of the elderly, can be compensated for by the use of large-faced clocks.
3. *Cognitive behavior*. Room doors (and floors) that are color-coded to demarcate important routes (within institutions or elsewhere) help older people ''map out'' their environment.
4. *Self-maintenance skills*. Bathroom facilities can be arranged to anticipate the physical limits of old age (such as a side-bar to hold onto instead of relying on an attendant or helping person to assist with certain toilet functions). Kitchen facilities can be designed for simple nontaxing use by individuals.
5. *Effective behavior*. The availability of hobbies, various other recreational activities, and ''unprogrammed thinking'' can enhance morale. Emphasis on too-active participation, however, is not necessarily beneficial. (Lawton notes that much effecting behavior is vicarious). Enjoyment can also be obtained by sitting and watching other, more active, people.[63]

Additional prosthetic features of especial importance for institutional environments include: (1) *prostheses for a sense of time*, such as numerous large calendars that clearly show the day, week, or season or that announce important social events. (2) *Prostheses that enhance the sense of self*, as evidenced by the provision of mirrors for client rooms and ample space in which to store personal objects and display family photographs and mementos. (3) *Prostheses that encourage staff-patient intermingling*. This can mean simply placing staff offices adjacent to patient space. (4) *Prostheses for vicarious social involvement*. This can be arranged by designing nursing homes and other institutions so that ward activity can be easily observed when people sit outside their rooms. This could be done by organizing client rooms in a semi-circle around a central activity space. (5) *Prostheses for autonomy.* Nursing home residents should be able to choose different ways of using their environment. This could be accomplished by providing individual rooms for privacy plus space where small groups of residents can sit outside their room doors and talk together. (6) *Prostheses for general social interaction.* Institutions could be designed so that corridors intersect. The probability of social interaction increases where pathways cross.

Optimal Environments and the "Best Fit" Idea

In keeping with the notion that human behavior is best understood as the product of the interaction between environmental forces and the unique characteristics of the individual, all people will not find the same environment equally beneficial to their growth, development, or general functioning. The stimulating urban environment that the physically able older person might enjoy exploring may be overwhelmingly stressful to a peer who is less physically competent. Institutional living that maximizes prosthetic design features may be perfect for some of the elderly but terribly stifling or dulling for others. The active older person who maintains a strong sense of inner resourcefulness may only need to be informed about activities available in the community in order to become a participant, but the aged individual who stresses the significance of fate, luck, or the influence of others, as opposed to one's own sense of initiative, may need to be motivated by an outreach worker in order to become involved in some community activity. Education or information about "what is out there" may not provide sufficient motivation to conquer fears of traveling to even the safest locations. The beneficial qualities of any environment depend on the psychological and constitutional characteristics of the individual that it contains.

Perhaps the best statement on the subject has been made by Nahemow and Lawton, who note that the older person functions best in a "moderately challenging environment."[64] Too much stimulation may be overwhelming and may lead to dysfunctional behavior (such as withdrawal), but too little stimulation is not challenging enough and can induce lethargy and encourage people to operate below their capacities. The moderately challenging environment is one that *best fits* the optimal functioning capacity of the person. We must always keep in mind, however, that what is moderately challenging for one older person may not be so for another. Those who work with the aged must consider both individual capacities and the challenge provided by the environment. Such thinking can lead to better design of activities and programs for the aged.

SOCIAL CHARACTERISTICS OF THE AGED

Who the aged are is defined, not only by biological processes, aspects of personality development, or cultural and environmental factors, but also by social characteristics, such as population distribution, income and educational levels, and living arrangements. In this section, we briefly survey some of these social characteristics of aging.

Demographics

According to the 1980 census, there are 25.5 million people over age 65 residing in the United States; this represents 11.3 percent of the U.S. population.

The 1977 National Center on Health Statistics (NCHS) report on a national nursing home survey indicates that there were 1.3 million people residing in qualified nursing facilities and facilities for intermediate care. Out of the 1.3 million, 1.1 million were over 65. This group is probably larger now, because most estimates indicate that about 5 percent of the over-65 population resides in nursing homes.

Breakdown by Age

Currently, 61 percent of the older population are between ages 65 and 74; 30 percent are between 75 and 84; and 9 percent are 85 and over.

Examination of the nursing-home population has shown the median age of residents to be 81 years. By age, the breakdown is: 1.4 percent of those 65 to 74, 6.8 percent of those 75 to 84, and 21.6 percent of those 85 and over reside in nursing homes.[65]

Increases in the elderly population are primarily the result of improvements in child care and disease prevention in early life. More people are surviving infancy and reaching adulthood. Although more people are living longer, nevertheless, expected increases in longevity, although substantial, are not spectacular.[66] It seems that life expectancy will be greatly increased only if certain medical breakthroughs are achieved. For example, it has been estimated that the elimination of death caused by cancer or stroke for persons aged 65 and over would increase their life expectancy by one and one-half years and that elimination of death caused by heart disease would add as much as five years. The greatest impact on longevity would come from elimination of the major cardiovascular and renal diseases. If this were achieved, ten years could be added to life expectancy at age 65.[67]

Two Older Populations

Because more people are reaching adulthood (because the death rate is gradually decreasing), we will soon have two groups of old people: the young-old and the old-old. For example, between 1940 and 1970, there was a 9 percent decrease in the proportion of the older population aged 65 through 74 years, and in the same period, the relative number of those aged 75 through 84 years increased from 25 percent to over 30 percent. In addition, the 85-plus portion of the population jumped from almost 4 percent of the aged in 1940 to 8 percent in 1970 and to 9 percent in 1982.[68]

The older population is itself aging. This redistribution of age groups may greatly affect our concepts of "normal" life stages. It suggests that we begin to view the postretirement years as a *transition* stage into old age, which (in turn) may carry implications for discovering new developmental tasks through leisure.[69]

Distribution of the Older Population by Sex

The ratio of older women to older men has changed radically since the turn of the century. Table 3–3 gives the number of females per 100 males aged 60 and over in the United States for the years 1900 and 1974.

TABLE 3–3. NUMBER OF FEMALES PER 100 MALES 60 YEARS AND OVER IN THE UNITED STATES IN 1900 AND 1974

Age	Females per 100 Males	
	1900	*1974*
TOTAL	97.0	133.8
60–64 years	95.3	114.1
65–74 years	95.7	130.1
75–84 years	101.0	160.9
85 years and over	125.4	202.1

Adapted from U.S. Department of Health, Education, and Welfare. Statistical Memo No. 31. *Publication (OHD) 75-20013. Washington, D.C.; May, 1975 (Table B. p. 3).*

The number of females per 100 males has increased dramatically since 1900. This trend is expected to continue through the year 2000. It is of interest that the greatest discrepancy between females and males appears in the older age categories. At age 85 and over, there were in 1974 more than two females for every male. By the year 2000, this ratio will also hold for the 75-plus category. Such trends obviously carry implications for female role definition, marital status, housing, and income policies. Projections for the future are shown in Table 3–4.

Income, Education, and Living Arrangements

Since there are currently some 26 million people over age 65 in the United States, the task of describing who the aged are might be easily subject to overgeneralization. Twenty-six million people are not, and cannot, be exactly alike. In fact, it appears that, as we grow older, individual differences are more likely to emerge.[70] However, by looking at such factors as income levels, educational levels, and living arrangements of the aged, we may better realize that the elderly do share some similarities. These factors remind us that the elderly do, in fact, experience a different quality of life from their younger counterparts.

In terms of living arrangements, one fact clearly stands out: The aged do not all

TABLE 3–4. CENSUS BUREAU PROJECTIONS FOR THE NUMBER OF ELDERLY IN SELECTED FUTURE YEARS: POPULATION (MILLIONS) IN AGE GROUP

Year	Age Group		
	55 Years and Above	*65 Years and Above*	*75 Years and Above*
1970	38.7	20.1	7.6
1980	45.6	24.5	9.1
1990	49.4	28.9	11.4
2000	53.5	30.6	13.5
2010	65.7	33.2	13.9
2020	79.5	42.8	15.4
2030	82.5	51.6	20.7
2040	84.8	50.3	24.2

United States Bureau of the Census, 1976.

live in nursing homes or institutions. Recent statistics indicate that only 5 percent of those over age 65 are institutionalized and that a large percentage of the noninstitutionalized aged are very active. Less than 1 percent of persons over age 65 are patients in mental hospitals, and current estimates indicate that less than 10 percent of those living in and outside of institutions have severe mental illness. The vast majority of those classified as older are therefore not particularly hindered by unusual forms of mental illness. Additional information on living arrangements indicates that older women are more likely than older men to live alone, due to the earlier death of their spouses.[71]

Older people have traditionally had less formal education than their younger counterparts. Recent estimates show that, on the average, older people have had more than four years less schooling than younger members of the population (aged 25 to 64).[72] This trend is rapidly changing, however, and in the near future, it is likely that older people will have as much formal education as our nation's youth, (perhaps even more, as a result of the rise in continuing education).

In terms of income, the aged comprise one of the poorest segments of our population. Recent statistics show that those 65 and over made up 14.6 percent of all poor in the United States, while 16.3 percent of all old people are poor, compared to 11.1 percent of people of all ages. Poverty is here defined by the poverty threshold, which is based on government standards and is tied to the consumer price index. This threshold has been defined as an income of $2,130 a year for a single person and $2,680 a year for a couple. In fact, it has been estimated that more than one-half of the elderly suffer significant economic deprivation.[73]

The problems associated with income among the elderly have entered into the realm of treatment modalities. To some, for example, the most powerful intervention that society can make in order to help the aged is to provide economic support. The importance of income is further reflected in the findings of a national sample of retirees, which revealed that the most significant determination of postretirement satisfaction was having an adequate income.[74]

REFERENCE NOTES

1. Sacher, G. A. Theory in gerontology. *Annual Review of Gerontology and Geriatrics*. New York: Springer, 1980, *1*, pp. 3–25.
2. Costa, P. T. & McCrae R. R. Still stable after all these years: Personality as a key to some issues in adulthood and old age. In P. E. Baltes & O. G. Brin (Eds.), *Life-span development and behavior*. New York: Academic Press, 1980, pp. 65–102.
3. Botwinick, J. *Aging and behavior*. New York: Springer, 1984, p. 144.
4. Buhler, C. *Der Menschliche Lebenslauf als Psychologisches Problem*. Leipzig: Herzel, 1933; 2nd ed., Gottingen: Verlag fuer Psychologie, 1959; Buhler, C. The curve of life as studies in biographies. *Journal of Applied Psychology*, 1953, *19*, 405–409; Buhler, C. Human life goals in the humanistic perspective. *Journal of Humanistic Psychology*, 1967, *7*, 36–52.
5. Buhler. *Human life goals in the humanistic perspective*, p. 49.
6. Ellenberger, H. F. *The discovery of the unconscious*. New York: Basic Books, 1970.
7. Jung, C. G. *Memories, dreams, reflections*. New York: Pantheon Books, 1963; Jung,

C. G. The stages of life, in *The collected works of C. G. Jung: Structure and dynamics of the psyche*, Vol. 8, (Trans., R.F.C. Hull). New York: Pantheon Books, 1960.
8. Guttman, D. Parenthood: A key to the comparative study of the life cycle. In N. Datan & L. H. Ginsberg (Eds.), *Life-span developmental psychology: Normative life crises*. New York: Academic Press, 1975.
9. Ellenberger, *The discovery of the unconscious*.
10. Jung. The stages of life, p. 20.
11. Erikson, E. H. Reflections on Dr. Borg's life cycle. *Daedalus*, 1976, *105*, 1–28.
12. Erikson, E. H. Identity and the life cycle. *Psychological Issues*, 1959, *I*, 98.
13. Erikson, Reflections on Dr. Borg's life cycle, p. 23.
14. Ibid., p. 23.
15. Peck, R. C. Psychological developments in the second half of life. In J. E. Anderson (Ed.), *Psychological aspects of aging*. Washington, D.C.: American Psychological Association, 1956.
16. Butler, R. M. Re-awakening interest. *Nursing homes*, 1961, *10*, 8–19.
17. Butler, R. M. & Lewis, M. I. *Aging and mental health*. St. Louis: C.V. Mosby, 1973.
18. Brink, T. L. *Geriatric psychotherapy*. New York: Human Sciences Press, 1977, pp. 181–182.
19. Ibid.
20. Botwinick, *Aging and behavior*.
21. Conte, H., Weiner, M. B., & Plutchik, R. Measuring death anxiety: Conceptual, psychometric, and factor-analytic aspects. *Journal of Personality and Social Psychology*, 1982, *43*(4), 775–785.
22. Pollak, J. M. Correlates of death anxiety. A review of empirical studies. *Omega*, 1980, *10*, 97–121.
23. Koocher, G. P., O'Malley, J. E., Foster, D., & Gogan, J. L. Death anxiety in normal children and adolescents. *Psychiatria Clinica*, 1976, *9*, 220–229.
24. Kubler-Ross, E. *On death and dying*. New York: Macmillan, 1969.
25. Kastenbaum, R. Is death a life crisis? In Datan & Ginsberg (Eds.), *Life-span developmental psychology: Normative life crises*. New York: Academic Press, 1975.
26. Kubler-Ross, *On death and dying*.
27. Kastenbaum, *Is death a life crisis?*
28. Clark, M. The anthropology of aging: A new area for studies of culture and personality. In B. L. Neugarten (Ed.), *Middle age and aging*. Chicago: The University of Chicago Press, 1968.
29. Birron, J. E., & Woodruff, D. S. Human development over the life span through education. In P. B. Baltes & K. W. Schaie (Eds.), *Life span developmental psychology: personality and socialization*. New York: Academic Press, 1973.
30. Bosse, R. & Ekerdt, D. J. Change in self-perception of leisure activities with retirement. *The Gerontologist*, 1981, *21*(6), 651–654.
31. Clark. *The anthropology of aging: A new area for studies of culture and personality*.
32. Clark, M. An anthropological view of retirement. In F. M. Carp (Ed.), *Retirement*. New York: Behavioral Publications, 1972.
33. Miller, S. J. The social dilemma of the aging leisure participant. In Neugarten (Ed.), Middle age and aging; Clark, An anthropological view of retirement.
34. Clark, *An anthropological view of retirement*.
35. Bennett, R. & Eckman, J. Attitudes toward aging: A critical examination of recent literature and implications for future research. In Eisdorfer & Lawton (Eds.), *The psychology of adult development and aging*.

36. Tuckman, J., & Lorge, I. Attitudes toward old people. *Journal of Social Psychology*, 1953, *37*, 249–260; Tuckman, J., & Lorge, I. The influence of changed directions on stereotypes about aging: before and after instructions. *Educational and Psychological Measurement*, 1954, *14*, 128–132; Tuckman, J. & Lorge, I. Attitude toward aging of individuals with experience with the aged. *Journal of Genetic Psychology*, 1958, *92*, 199–204, American Psychological Association, 1973.
37. Lutsky, N. S. Attitudes toward old age and elderly persons. *Annual Review of Gerontology and Geriatrics*, 1980, *1*, 287–336; Wingard, J. A. Measures of attitudes toward the elderly: A statistical reevaluation of comparability. *Experimental Aging Research*, 1980, *6*, 299–313.
38. Wingard, J. A., Heath, R., & Himelstein, S. A. The effects of contextual variations on attitudes toward the elderly. *Journal of Gerontology*, 1982, *33*(4), 474–482.
39. Axelrod, S., & Eisdorfer, C. Attitudes toward old people: An empirical analysis of the stimulous group validity of the Tuckman–Lorge questionnaire. *Journal of Gerontology*, 1961, *16*, 75–80.
40. Tuckman, J., & Lorge, I. Attitudes toward old people. *Journal of Social Psychology*, 1953, *37*, 249–260.
41. Kogan, N., & Shelton, F. C. Beliefs about "old people": A comparative study of older and younger samples. *The Journal of Genetic Psychology*, 1962, *100*, 93–111.
42. Bennett, R., & Eckman, J. Attitudes toward aging: Critical examination of recent literature and implications for future research. In C. Eisdorfer and M. P. Lawton (Eds.), *The psychology of adult development and aging*. Washington, D.C.: American Psychological Association, 1973.
43. Wingard, Heath, & Himelstein, The effects of contextual variations on attitudes toward the elderly.
44. Austin, D. R., Attitudes toward old age: A hierarchical study. *The Gerontologist*, 1985, *25*(4), 431–434.
45. Baker, R. R., Attitudes of health care providers toward elderly patients with normal aging and disease-related symptoms. *The Gerontologist*, 1984, *24*(5), 543–545.
46. Okum, M. A., & Divesta, F. J. Cautiousness in adulthood as a function of age and instructions. *Journal of Gerontology*, 1976, *31*, 571–576; Botwinick, J. *Aging and behavior*, 1973, New York: Springer.
47. J. Botwinick, *Aging and behavior*.
48. Wallach, M., & Kogan, N. Aspects of judgment and decision making interrelations and changes with age. *Behavioral Science*, 1961, *6*, 23–36.
49. Ibid., p. 27.
50. Botwinick, J. Cautiousness in advanced age. *Journal of Gerontology*, 1966, *21*, 347–353.
51. Botwinick, J. Disinclination to venture response versus cautiousness in responding. *Journal of Genetic Psychology*, 1969, *115*, 55–62.
52. Brok, A. J. *Issues in leisure relevant to counseling and applied human development*. Paper presented at the 83rd annual meeting of the American Psychological Association, Chicago, 1975.
53. Brok, A. J. & Westcott, W. *Age and sex differences in free time interests: An exploratory inquiry*. Paper presented at the 46th annual meeting of the Eastern Psychological Association, New York, 1975.
54. Schaie, K. W. Translations in gerontology from lab to life: Intellectual functioning. *American Psychologist*, 1974, *29*, 802–807.
55. Ibid., p. 804.

56. Gottesman, L., Quarterman, C. E., & Cohn, G. M. Psychosocial treatment of the aged. In C. Eisdorfer & M. Lawton (Eds.), *The psychology of adult development and aging*. Washington, D.C.: American Psychological Association, 1973. Nahemow, L., & Lawton, M. P. Toward an ecological theory of adaptation and aging. In H. Proshansky, W. H. Ittelson, & L. G. Rivlin (Eds.), *Environmental Psychology, 2nd ed*. New York: Holt, Rinehart, & Winston, 1976.
57. Steinfeld, E. H. Ecology of aging. In *An instructor's handbook for the development of a basic course in gerontology*. Syracuse, N.Y.: Syracuse University All-University Gerontology Center, 1975.
58. Gottesman, Quarterman, & Cohn, *Psychosocial treatment of the aged.*
59. Steinfeld, *Ecology of aging.*
60. Ittelson, W. H., Proshansky, M. H., Rivlin, L. G., & Winkel, G. H. *An introduction to environmental psychology*. New York: Holt, Rinehart, & Winston, 1974.
61. Ibid.
62. Nahemow, L. & Kogan, L. S. *Reduced fare for the elderly*. New York: Mayor's Office for the Aging, 1971.
63. Lawton, M. P. *Social and structural aspects of prosthetic environments for older people*. Paper presented at the Third Annual Institute on Man's Adjustment in a Complex Environment, Veterans Administration Hospital, Brecksville, Ohio, June, 1968; Lawton, M. P. Some beginnings of an ecological psychology of old age. In J. F. Wohwill & D. H. Caison (Eds.), *Environment and the social sciences:* Washington, D.C.: American Psychological Association, 1972.
64. Nahemow and Lawton, *Toward an ecological theory of adaptation and aging*, p. 319.
65. Teresi, J., Holmes, M., & Holmes, D. *Sheltered living environments for the elderly*. Paper prepared for the Administration on Aging, Office of Human Development Services, August, 1982.
66. U.S. Department of Health, Education, and Welfare. *Statistical memo no. 31*, Publication (OHD) 75-20013. Washington, D.C., May 1975.
67. Brotman, H. B. *Who are the aging?* In E.W. Busse & E. Pfeiffer (Eds.), *Mental illness in later life*. Washington, D.C.: American Psychiatric Association, 1973.
68. Teresi, J., Holmes, M., & Holmes, D. *Sheltered living environments for the elderly*.
69. Brok, *Issues in leisure relevant to counseling and applied human development*.
70. Brotman, *Who are the aging?*
71. Gottesman, Quarterman, and Cohn, *Psychosocial treatment of the aged;* Palmore, E. Social factors in mental illness of the aged. In Busse & Pfeiffer (Eds.), *Mental illness in later life*. Brotman, *Who are the aging?* American Psychiatric Association, 1973.
72. Brotman, *Who are the aging?*
73. U.S. Department of Health, Education, and Welfare. *Facts and figures on older Americans*, No. 11, Publication (OHD) 75-20012. Washington, D.C., February 1975; Hume, S. *Basic course in gerontology*. Albany, N.Y.: School of Social Welfare, State University of New York at Albany, 1975.
74. Gottesman, Quarterman, & Cohn, *Psychosocial treatment of the aged*; Barfield, R., & Morgan, J. *Early retirement*. Ann Arbor, Mich.: Survey Research Center, 1968.

PART II

The Institutionalized Aged

4

The Institutionalized Aged

Surveys have shown that some 814,000 persons over age 65 are living in institutions—only about 5 percent of the country's older people. Approximately one in seven of these was in a psychiatric facility; almost all of the rest were in nursing homes.[1] Studies show that the person who does enter an institution in later life is generally one who has been *chronically marginal;* that is, has not been able to cope adequately with the outside world through existing support systems, such as family. In caring for elderly patients who are considering placement in a nursing home, Terry L. Brink, Ph.D., advises alert physicians to first "inform yourself of the alternatives to institutionalization," noting that "patients treated at home tend to recover faster" and are "less likely to develop the mental confusion fostered by the featureless routine of institutional living."[2]

These marginal people are alone and isolated. Although they constitute but a small segment of today's elderly, it is on them that the commonly held stereotypes about aging are based. It is such stereotyping that makes aging itself increasingly harder to accept as a normative process. In fact, there are those who regard aging as a disability. In this section, we shall focus on that 5 percent of the institutionalized minority for whom aging *is* a disability.

INSTITUTIONALIZATION

Nursing homes, like mental hospitals or prisons, are *total institutions*—"places of residence where a large number of like-situated individuals together lead an enclosed, formally administered round of life."[3] When one enters an institution, mastery or command over his or her world is disrupted; so much so that Goffman calls those who are institutionalized "inmates."

There occurs what Goffman terms a *mortification of self,* in the form of the loss of roles, of personal property, or even of one's full name. There may be a disidentifying process, such as the belief that "I don't really belong here." This disidentification may be a reaction against "contaminative exposure"—exposure to others less competent. In the nursing home, we must anticipate this reaction from an alert resident who is exposed to a resident who is confused and regressed. We also expect this as a reaction to the commonly held stereotype of the nursing home as a place to wait for death. These concepts may partially explain why residents appear so detached from one another.

In every institution, there occurs a *looping process*: everything is fed back into everything else. Dress and manners, for example, are under constant scrutiny, as are staff and residents' conversations. The result is maximum visibility and minimum privacy. In addition, there exists in every institution a "caste system," an authoritarian staff class constantly doling out discipline to the residents. In reality, institutions are generally run according to staff convenience.

In an article emphasizing the responsibility of physicians in the care of the institutionalized elderly, Brink recommends rehabilitation rather than the use of tranquilizers, plus careful checking for adverse drug reactions when drugs are indicated. If a patient's care is inadequate in any nursing home, he urges vigilant physicians to complain, filing protests with the facility's director or with appropriate state and local agencies, or even advising the family to relocate the patient.[4]

The sociological consequences of institutionalization have been aptly described.[5] It is no wonder that prolonged institutionalization is said to cause *desocialization*. Psychologically, an *institutional neurosis* has been described as a syndrome characterized by apathy, lack of initiative, lack of expression of feelings of resentment, lack of interest in the future, and deterioration of personal habits.[6] It is not surprising that many an institutionalized person is starved for some form of meaningful interaction that would improve the quality of his life.

Isolation

Loneliness, isolation, and desolation are often the destiny of the elderly. While this is recognized as true for the institutionalized elderly, recent reports indicate a direct link between the possibility of living alone and becoming mentally disabled, even for those living in the community.[7] Conversely, when there is social interaction, as between neighbors, this likelihood is much reduced.

Isolation, as distinguished from loneliness, is the deprivation of social contact and content, while loneliness is a psychological state within the person. Stressing that social interaction, as a means of fending off or even reversing isolation, needs to be encouraged, Bennett states that "for those aged who are isolated, there is a need for resocialization, which is particularly important to older persons at points of death and/or institutionalization."[8] The concentrated efforts of researchers continually assessing the impact of isolation on the aged are underway. Even more critical are the intervention programs aimed at reducing the isolation of the elderly in institutional settings.

Incontinence

A condition that brings with it the wish to be isolated, along with the effect of shame or embarrassment, is incontinence of bladder and bowel. Who wants to be in the presence of others when there is constant worry about the possibility of an "accident"? The elderly are often heard to say, "I want to live only as long as I have my wits about me and I don't soil myself. If that's gone, life is not worth living." Incontinence is the ultimate embarrassment.

There are many causes for incontinence; provided that physical problems are ruled out, there is much that staff in the institution can do to prevent and ease this problem. For instance, identifying patients on diuretics and seeing that such medications are administered no later than 10 A.M. can do much to alleviate nighttime incontinence. Old bones don't move so fast, and providing a bedside commode can help someone who cannot make it to the bathroom in time. Rooms should have a nightlight so that a patient can see the way to the bathroom. In turn, the bathroom should be identified with a symbol on the door so that it can be distinguished from other doorways in the room or corridor. A bedpan or urinal should be within easy reach and should be emptied when it has been used. But patients don't have to bother using bedpans when their contents spill into the bed anyway after accumulating over an eight-hour shift! Call bells should be answered as quickly as possible, since weak muscles may not be able to maintain control if help doesn't come soon enough.

While we may not be able to "cure" incontinence, we can control the loss of dignity associated with this condition. Sensitive care, recognizing that shame can be reduced and human dignity maintained in the patient, will offer its own rewards.

WHO IS THE NURSING-HOME PATIENT?

The median age of nursing-home patients is 81 years. The breakdown by age of those residing in nursing homes is: 1.4 percent of the 65 to 74 age group, 6.8 percent of the 75 to 84 age group, and 21.6 percent of the 85-plus group.[9] Seventy-one percent of nursing home patients are women, partially because they live longer than men and partially because women are more likely to remain widowed and alone. From 60 to 80 percent are poor, even though they may not have been poor before they were old. The vast majority have more than one chronic physical ailment. Nineteen percent have severe hearing defects, and approximately 12 percent have severe visual impairments. Only one-sixth of all nursing-home patients are confined to bed. It is estimated that one-half of those elderly who are confined to nursing homes suffer from mental disorders or senility.[10]

Chronic Brain Syndrome and the Institutionalized Aged

The layperson calls it *senility*. The professional calls it *chronic brain syndrome*, *organic brain syndrome*, *organic mental state*, *senile dementia*, *dementia of the Alzheimer type*, or *senile psychosis*. Although dementia of the Alzheimer type characterizes 50 percent of all senile dementia, all of these terms are likely to be applied to a large percentage of aging patients in long-term-care facilities. These residents suffer various physical, cognitive, and emotional impairments and exhibit symptoms of deterioration such as confusion, disorientation, faulty recent memory, emotional lability, indifference, poor interpersonal relationships, and apathy. It is estimated that at least 50 percent of all patients 65 and over in long-term-care facilities are suffering from some type of dementia. Also, many behaviors that merely reflect individual differences in personality are often labeled "senile," sometimes with tragic consequences.

Despite various physiological investigations and therapeutic attempts, the etiology of the symptoms (other than age) still remains unclear; however, the contributions of sensory impairment and social isolation have been recognized.[11] Monotony, boredom, and isolation often create similar symptoms in younger subjects; in older subjects, these same conditions tend to heighten the symptoms of organic deterioration.[12]

No longer is there generalized espousal of the attitude that nothing can be done for the aging institutionalized person, for progress has been made in the alleviation of some of the symptoms of senility. Physical interventions have been tried, sometimes with limited success, but with success nonetheless. Trials have included anticoagulation therapy, hyperoxygenation, and vitamin B_{12} administration. Now recognized is the fact that elderly people suffering from such treatable disorders as nutritional deficiencies, tumors, anemia, depression, hyperthyroidism, and other metabolic problems are sometimes dismissed and neglected, having been mistakenly classified as "hopelessly senile."[13]

In the affective domain, it has been demonstrated that, even in very deteriorated, very old patients, intensified sensory input produces significant behavioral changes.[14] It is currently recognized that senile symptoms may sometimes be behavioral manifestations of maladjustment, neuroticism, anxiety, and lack of ego strength resulting from a decline in participation in the environment and induced sensory deprivation. In fact, certain memory losses have been found to be selective. It has been suggested, therefore, that some senile symptoms are reversible.[15] If there is no appropriate intervention, however, senility becomes a vicious spiral, as shown in Figure 4–1.

Drugs

Much as senility, both real and misdiagnosed, can create apathy and its own dead-end spiral, so too can the problem of drugs administered to the older patient.

The older person living in a nursing home is very dependent upon the personnel serving her or him. These personnel, though they may be well-meaning, may be more concerned about making their jobs easier than about the welfare of their patients. One of the sad results of this may be the administration of excessive or inappropriate drugs.

Iatrogenic, or doctor-induced, disease is a reality today. The pattern is well-known: At home, people often take a combination of medications given to them by several different physicians. In addition, they may take a variety of over-the-counter

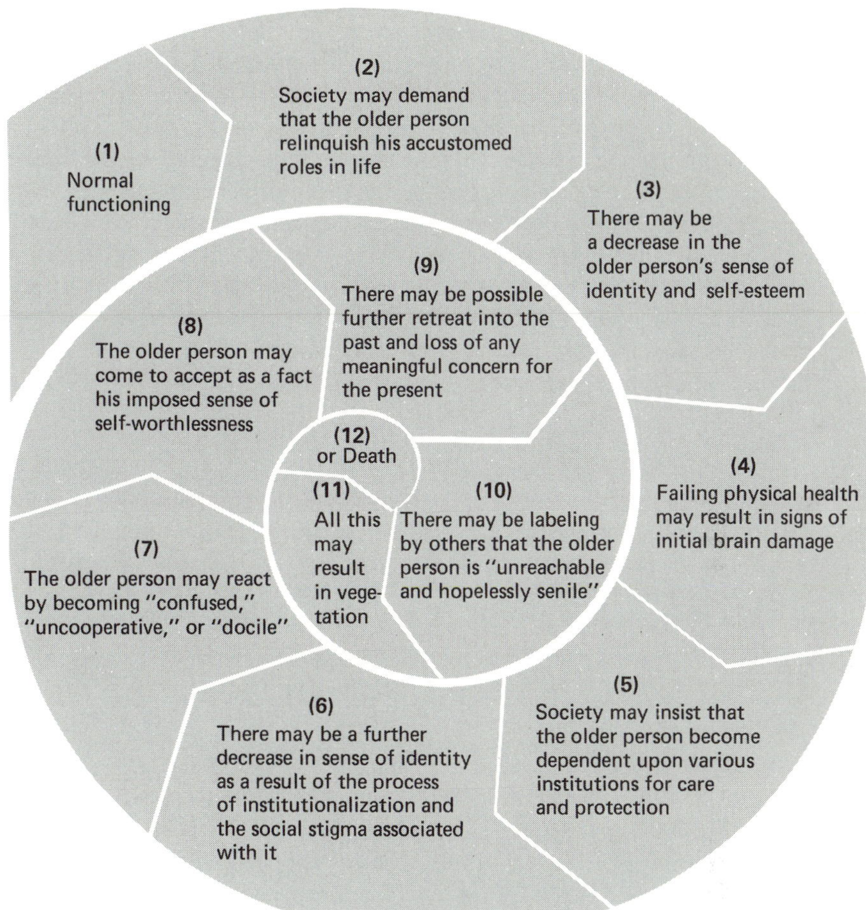

Figure 4–1. The spiral of senility. The patient may not go through all the stages shown nor in the order shown; however, all stages have been observed clinically in different patients at different times. Note that a consistently observed pattern in the spiral is the progressive decrease in self-esteem, ending in death. *(From Barnes, E. K., Sack, A., & Shore, H. Guidelines to treatment approaches.* Gerontologist, *1973,* 13, *513–527.)*

medications. Upon entering the nursing home or long-term-care facility, the patient may not be completely evaluated by a geriatrician. Instead of a thorough evaluation—i.e., physical and psychological exams and complete blood work, including blood levels of drugs currently being taken—orders may be written to continue the regime that the person is currently on. It has been suggested that the average older person in a nursing home may receive as many as seven different drugs each day.[16] Medications may be re-ordered month after month without a re-examination of the patient. Since approximately 40 percent of all drugs prescribed are for analgesics, sedatives, and tranquilizers, it is of interest that over half of these prescriptions are for tranquilizers alone, the "chemical straitjacket."[17]

As we know, aging brings with it physiological changes that affect the clearance and utilization of drugs by the body. The ratio of fat to muscle increases, and drugs that bind up with fat rather than with protein may rise to dangerously high levels in a rapid fashion. The amount of time necessary for clearance by the kidneys changes, as does the time needed for the circulation and absorption of drugs throughout the body.[18] In addition, many drugs commonly ordered for the elderly may have adverse side effects, such as confusion, restlessness, change in gait, or irritability of the soma and psyche. Muscle relaxants relax many muscles, not just the particular muscle needing attention! As a result, a patient may have bowel and bladder changes unrelated to actual physical deterioration.

As one geriatric nurse told us:[19]

> Our older population in the United States is heavily medicated. This is true especially among the poor, who are the ones who wind up in the institution. These are the people who, before institutionalization, tended to go to many doctors and hospital clinics with their multiple ailments. This necessitated their being cared for by a number of practitioners with varying specialties. Each of these specialists prescribed medications to address the problem for which the patient was consulting him or her. The patient may not remember or may not consider it important that she or he is taking a number of other medications. Together, the potential for drug interaction, and occasional duplication, is high.

As may be predicted, outdated and old medications are not thrown away; they are often saved in order to be taken when the patient has a symptom that he or she thinks will be helped by that particular drug. This pattern may follow the patient into the institution. Over-the-counter drugs may be brought to the patient by family members or well-intentioned friends. Such drugs may be traded among patients. And drugs are often palmed (pretending to take one when given by the nurse, but in reality, stored for later use).

We are not suggesting that drugs should never be administered; we are suggesting that they should be properly monitored. Where proper monitoring exists, great benefit can take place for the person who is our primary concern—the patient. This was shown in a study comparing two groups of nursing-home patients. Both groups were living in intermediary-care facilities. The first group was followed by local physicians, while the second was assigned to a geriatric medical team consisting of a geriatrician and a physician's assistant. After seven months, it was found that the first group received six medications per patient prescription, while the second received two. Although the number of medications was lower for those assigned to the geriatric team, the number of medical visits (by patients to doctors) increased, the first group reaching 0.5 visits per month and the second, 1.7. The rate of mortality, hospitalization, and transfer to a skilled nursing facility was markedly reduced in the second group.[20] Proper drug monitoring and good care appear to have had their effects. Most important, when these take place, the older person is not reduced to a shell of her or his former self by chemicals instead of his or her own life force.

In considering drugs for the patient, staff members have the obligation to look at the overall picture. Evaluating a patient's drug profile with the aid of the pharmacist, monitoring for drug interaction and side effects, and sharing this information with medical staff and other team personnel are essential. Alternate therapies, such as massage, heat, physiotherapy, and diet, should also be explored.

Self-esteem

The sense of self that we develop in early life becomes a basic part of our personality and of our ability to adapt to our environment. Self-esteem builds from one's own achievements, activities, and sense of mastery. This sense of self is an important factor in determining the degree to which such problems as rejection, failure, physical illness, and stress can be tolerated. With aging and its accompanying stresses, such as role loss, physical illness, and financial insecurity, there is decreased opportunity for the continued sense of mastery that is an essential ingredient of self-esteem.

This may be particularly true for the institutionalized aging person, because the institutional complex may not lend itself to activities or personal interactions that build and help maintain one's self-esteem. In addition, choices within our institutions are limited, so that one is given less opportunity to exercise one's sense of self. Mastery of the environment is often not encouraged. Instead, the institution pushes for the person to be the "good" patient—the patient who will show little incentive or initiative and who will make little trouble for the staff. This "model patient" often suffers from a decreased sense of worth. It is no wonder that depression, with its accompanying feelings of worthlessness, is the most prevalent psychological problem found in older people.

Depression

Depression may vary from feeling low to complete withdrawal or even suicide. Older people experiencing depression often state that, during such times, they feel discouraged, worried, or disgusted with their own uselessness. Often, they make statements such as "There is just no reason to go on living" or "I would welcome death."

Depression in the institutionalized older patient may often be masked and so may go unnoticed. This masking may be expressed by the patient's verbal listing of a host of somatic complaints. This is due, in part, to the fact that aging persons in our society are "allowed" to be sick and are often reinforced for this by the attention that they receive from staff and others. Depressed persons may then have a host of people "fussing" over them only as long as they verbalize feelings of being ill. If they state that they are depressed, others may move away from them without tuning into what could be behind the depression, such as feelings of anger turned inward or, most common, a type of mourning related to loss. Losses and decline are common in old age. The older person has less physical vitality, less mental agility, and less overall stamina. Of great impact are losses of loved persons. These losses contribute greatly to feelings of social isolation and loneliness. Feelings of loneliness are heightened by a move into an impersonal institution. Along with this may also come distortions in body image.

Such losses are currently recognized as a sense of "loss of self." Elderly persons who, throughout life, have placed little value on their own selves are vulnerable to depression in their later years, for "it is this response to the experience of failing parts of the self which produces the observed phenomenon of depression."[21] Whether the losses are primarily experienced as losses of failing parts of the self or as the loss of loved ones through death, "these losses contribute greatly to feelings of social isolation and loneliness."

Body Image

Closely related to lack of self-esteem and to depression are distortions of body image. These relate to misconceptions of one's sexual identity, one's size, one's strength, and one's beauty: "I am too short for anyone to love me," "I am ugly," "I am weak." These distortions or devaluations are not a function of aging per se, but rather, are a compilation of earlier experiences—past successes or failures, good or bad health, affection or neglect, love or dislike.

In a series of studies concerned with measuring the body image of six groups—four geriatric and two younger groups, with an overall age range of from 18 to 90 years—one of the oldest groups, with a mean age of 83 and residing in a home for the aged, scored lowest on indices measuring body worries and body discomforts, with a younger group residing in a mental hospital scoring the highest.[22] In a study of body image, as related to assigned dollar values for hypothetically lost body parts, there was no significant relationship between age and the dollar value placed either on individual parts or on the average for all body parts. Again, psychiatric patients placed significantly less value on their bodies than did persons who did not have psychiatric disorders, regardless of age. Together, these findings imply that, by itself, advanced age plays a less prominent role in impaired body image than do psychiatric status and environmental factors, such as lack of stimulation. Further studies also tend to support this implication.[23]

Sensory Deprivation

We are becoming more and more aware that people require, not only stimulation, but also varied sensory input for the maintenance of normal, adaptive behavior. Initial experiments attesting to this were conducted at McGill University in 1953. McGill students were paid $20 a day to remain in an environment that induced sensory deprivation. Despite the high rate of pay, subjects could not remain in that environment more than two to three days. During the experiment, much restlessness and emotional lability were observed, and after the experiment was over, students reported that they had had disturbances in visual, auditory, and perceptual spheres, as well as hallucinations, during the experiment. These data seemed to provide direct support for an intense dependence on one's environment that had not been previously suspected. Once someone is placed in an environment that lacks stimulation, a form of psychological "suspended animation" appears to take place.[24]

Both anatomical structure and optimal behavioral functioning require changes in external stimulation. It has been suggested that "no dramatic changes take place in the brain with aging when, and *only when*, stimulation is maintained.[25] Even in persons with *no* noticeable tissue damage, the deprivation of sensory stimuli can lead to bizarre behaviors, including hallucinations, delusions, depression, etc. Where deprivation is of a long-term nature, the person may become chronically impaired."[26]

In linking sensory deprivation experiments to aging, a study was performed in Australia involving sensory stimulation for treatment of what is termed senile dementia. Results of this study seem to confirm the fact that senile dementia may be only partially influenced by actual pathological changes occurring in the brain; it may be largely influenced by the sensory deprivation that accompanies the disease. This deprivation may be the result mainly of decreased social interaction. The authors of the study suggest that environmental stimulation may either slow down or, at times, reverse this process. Lack of stimulation may therefore be another contributing factor to chronic brain syndrome, perhaps one that could possibly be reduced by various intervention strategies.[27]

SOCIAL INTERACTION

While intervention strategies, described in the following chapters, are crucial for the well-being of the elderly nursing-home patient, so too is a form of bonding that we often neglect to recognize: friendships in the nursing home. We take for granted that living in the community affords us friends. We live independently and can make arrangements to call friends, see friends, make new friends, or restrict friendships that do not seem to be working. We act voluntarily and make decisions on our own. Although institutions have restrictions, people do not have to inevitably withdraw from social interaction once they enter a nursing home. Research has shown that key factors involving the formation of friendships between nursing-home patients were the resident's lucidity, the ability to communicate, and vision.[28] Outside-world bonding is often based upon similarities of social class, but this is not the case with nursing-home patients. They socialize across ethnic, religious, and social-class lines.

According to these studies, what was dominant in the formation of these friendships was location. Lucid patients who shared a room became friends if each was lucid and had his or her "senses." Although sight and mobility were important, hearing was less so, since total or partial deafness can be overcome by gesturing to that person, by shouting, or by communicating in other ways. Unlike community living, when friendships are often made with someone a good deal older or younger than oneself, the research suggests that, in the nursing home, age acts as the motivator for friendship.

While the nursing-home world offers restrictions, it may not be the "closed system" that it appears to be. It can contain a lively social world. Intimacy, the ability to touch another (concretely and in the abstract sense), remains a human need for all of our lives. Patients stripped of other roles, such as worker, spouse, or even parent, can still be friends. The friendship role is directly linked to patient morale. Workers should be aware that the nursing home need not be a "dead end," socially speaking, and that, despite its restrictions, the nursing home may offer possibilities for new friendships and new ways of living.

REFERENCE NOTES

1. Gottesman, L. E., Quarterman, C. E., & Cohn, G. M. Psychosocial treatment of the aged. In C. Eisdorfer & M. Lawton, *The psychology of adult development and aging*. Washington, D.C.: American Psychological Association, 1973.
2. Brink, T. L. Physician's responsibility for nursing home patients. *Journal of the National Medical Association*, 1977, *69*, 738.
3. Goffman, E. *Asylums*. New York: Anchor Books, 1961, p. 1.
4. Brink, Physician's responsibility for nursing home patients, p. 738.
5. Ibid.
6. Zusman, J. Some explanations of the changing appearance of psychotic patients. *International Journal of Psychiatry*, 1967, *4*, 216–237.
7. Magaziner, J. Living alone and psychopathology among the aged: neighborhood density as a protective factor. *The Gerontologist*, October 1982, *22*(5), 106.
8. Bennett, R. *Aging, isolation, and resocialization*. New York: Van Nostrand Reinhold Co., 1980.
9. Weiner, M. B., Teresi, J., & Streich, C. *Old people are a burden, but not my parents*. Englewood-Cliffs, N.J.: Prentice-Hall, Inc., 1983.
10. Butler, R. *Why survive? Being old in America*. New York: Harper & Row, 1975; Haggarty, A. D., The role of the long-term care facility. In M. Mitchel (Ed.), *A practical guide to long-term care and health services administration*. Greenvale, N.Y.: Panel Publishers, 1973.
11. Alexander, D. A. Senile dementia: a changing perspective. *British Journal of Psychiatry*, 1972, *121*, 207–214.
12. Loew, C. A., & Silverstone, B. M. A program of intensified stimulation and response facilitations for the senile aged. *The Gerontologist*, 1971, *11* 341–347.
13. Weiner, Teresi, & Streich, *Old people are a burden, but not my parents*.
14. Ibid.
15. Oberleder, M. Crisis therapy in mental breakdown of the aging. *The Gerontologist*, 1970, *10*, 111–114.
16. Sherwood, S., Mor, V., & Gutkin, C. A nationwide survey of domicilliary care for the aged: domicilliary care clients and the facilities in which they reside. National Institute for the Aging, 1981.
17. Ibid.
18. Steffi, B. M. *Handbook of Gerontological Nursing*. New York: Van Nostrand Reinhold Co., 1984.
19. Ben-Or, Rita. R.N., M.A. Deputy Director, Field Operations, Human Development Association. Personal communication.
20. Sorem, K., & Portnoi, V. Decreased rate of poly-pharmacy, hospitalization and mortality by geriatric medical team involvement in a nursing home. *The Gerontologist*, October, 1982, *22*(5), 21. (Abstract)
21. Weiner, M. B., Aging as ongoing adaptation to loss. In M. Tallmer et al., (Eds.), *The life-threatened elderly*. New York: Columbia University Press, 1984.
22. Plutchik, R., Weiner, M. B., & Conte, H. Studies of body image I: body worries and body discomforts. *Journal of Gerontology*, 1971, *26*, 344–350.
23. Plutchik, R., Conte, H., & Weiner, M. B. Studies of body image II: dollar values of body parts. *Journal of Gerontology*, 1973, *28*, 89–91; Plutchik, R., Conte, H., & Weiner, M. B. Studies of body image III: body feelings as measured by the semantic differential. *International Journal of Aging and Human Development*, 1973, *4*, 378–380.

24. Bexton, W. H., Heron, W., & Scott, T. H. Effects of decreased variation in the sensory environment. *Canadian Journal of Psychology*, 1954, *8*, 70–76.
25. Hussian, R. A. *Geriatric Psychology*. New York: Van Nostrand Reinhold Co., 1981, p. 135.
26. Ibid.
27. Bower, H. M. Sensory deprivation with aged: sensory stimulation and the treatment of senile dementia. *Experta Medica–Gerontology and Geriatrics*, 1968, *2*, 352.
28. Retsinas, J., & Garrity, P. Nursing home friendships. *The Gerontologist*, 1985, *25*(4), 376–381.

5

Rehabilitation: The Stepladder Approach

INTERVENTION STRATEGIES

There are so many psychosocial rehabilitative strategies, such as activities therapy, music therapy, drama therapy, poetry therapy, body movement therapy, and art therapy—so many that it is almost like alphabet soup! And workers who have a wide range of skills and of educational and experiential backgrounds use various techniques. Despite this diversity, however, all techniques share certain characteristics: (1) psychosocial stimulation, (2) opportunities for social interaction, and (3) opportunities for positive reinforcement related to growth and achievements. All are necessary ingredients of comprehensive care and may mitigate against the negative effects of institutionalization.

All of the therapies mentioned above, as well as others not listed, may be appropriate to patients who are considered to be fairly intact. (These therapies will be discussed later.) They are generally led by fairly specialized personnel. They may also be used in conjunction with each other and with a wide variety of modalities, as shown in Figure 5–1.

The techniques that we shall focus on here and in the chapters to follow—sensory training, reality orientation, and remotivation—are geared especially toward the more regressed, less intact patient. (It may be recalled that one-half of all nursing home patients have some form of mental disorder or senility.) These techniques are also to be used sequentially so that, when each is successfully completed, it leads to the next. We have labeled this the *stepladder approach*.

The Stepladder Approach to Rehabilitation

The stepladder approach can be used to match treatment modalities to the various levels of patient functioning. A very regressed patient is assigned to a basic treatment technique and then is moved up the ladder; that is, is assigned to successively

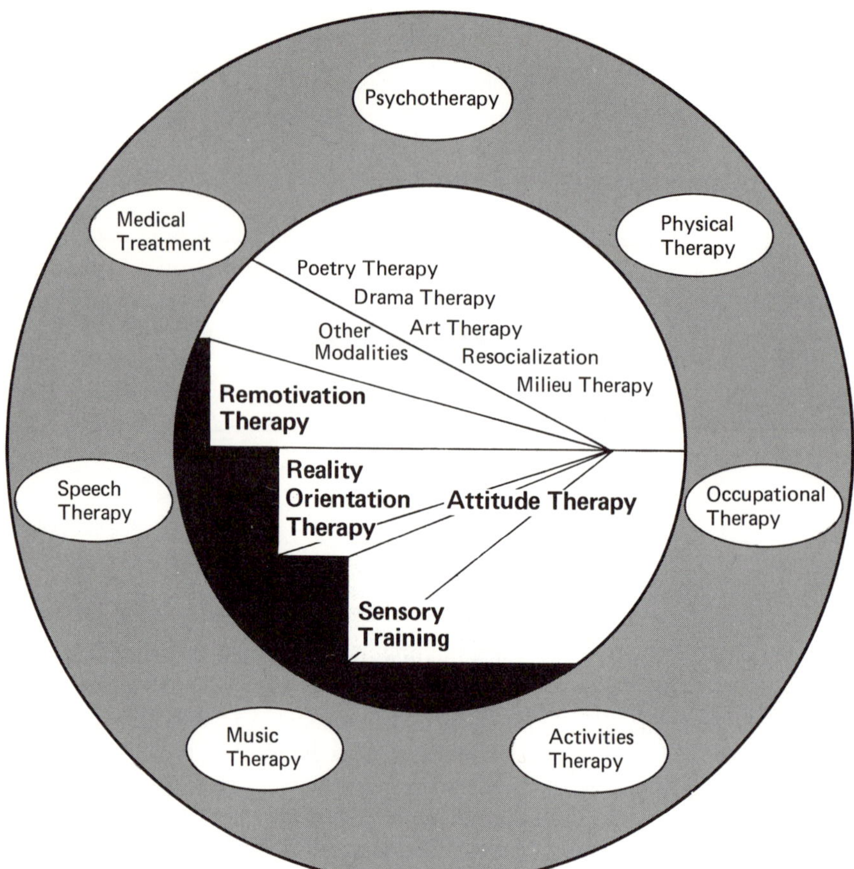

Figure 5–1. Rehabilitation is a many-faceted concept, with various interventions used simultaneously.

more complex techniques once he or she has experienced success on these lower levels.

Since chronic-brain-syndrome patients are often on a progressively downhill course, success may be minimal. In fact, there may be regression. In general, however, it has been clinically observed that patients are able to progress from one step to another.

Before looking at each technique in detail, we offer a brief description of each:

Sensory Training. Sensory training is a structured group/individual experience that involves all five senses. It is used with the regressed older person who shows an inability to interact with the environment. Its goal is to bring this individual back in touch with the surroundings by providing varied stimuli to improve the patient's response to the environment.

Reality Orientation. Reality orientation is a structured, common-sense behavioral approach to rehabilitating acutely or moderately confused patients to their immediate surroundings. It is a means of structuring the environment 24 hours a day so that staff can intervene appropriately and consistently with each confused person. This interaction may either prevent confusion or assist a confused person to regain an awareness of his or her "own identity and the concrete, existing realities in the surrounding environment."[1] The goal is to help the confused to relearn basic information about themselves and their environment in order to improve their awareness of time, place, and person.

Remotivation Therapy. Remotivation therapy is a structured program of group discussion that encourages patients to take renewed interest in their surroundings by focusing their attention on the simple, objective features of everyday life through a single relearning process.

These three techniques are a basic core of programs for patients who are less intact than others and who are unable to benefit sufficiently from the full range of program offerings. As a result of participation in these specialized, highly structured group programs, social interaction skills may be improved, and increased participation in other activities may become possible.

MATCHING PATIENTS TO TREATMENTS: A "BEST FIT" CONCEPT

Which kind of patient is best suited to which technique? Understanding this ensures that the technique most suited to an individual patient at a given time will be the one assigned. Matching patients to a particular technique or therapy may be redone at several points.

The Severely Regressed Patient: The First Step

Some patients appear to be more regressed because they are apathetic and withdrawn. Such a person often spends most of the time in his or her room or seeming to be asleep in an upright position during the day and is relatively inattentive to surroundings. Staff may refer to this patient as being "pretty much out of things." It may be that this behavior is a result of organic processes, an environment devoid of stimulation, or both factors. The end result, however, is that the patient appears relatively inactive and uninvolved.

If we take a developmental approach, we can see that this person would benefit most from sensory input. For example, the infant requires a great deal of stroking, caressing, and cuddling early in life. Although the geriatric patient is not to be infantilized, at the same time, he or she may require the same kinds of "stroking" as a result of the circumstances of these later years. Not having recently experienced much touching or interaction with others, the elderly may now require this sensory input. Stroking and reinforcement for alertness are crucial to the patient.

The older resident who is defined as being relatively regressed is a likely candidate for the first technique in the stepladder approach: sensory training. In order to determine if a patient best fits into this category, staff should confer with those most in contact with this person in order to obtain a general evaluation. If there is a designated team leader, as is the case in many facilities, this team leader would assign the patient to the modality of sensory training.

The Moderately Regressed Patient: The Second Step

The elderly person appropriate for this technique is one who has a good deal of difficulty in the cognitive sphere, tending to be confused and disoriented about time, place, and person. This may be the chronic-brain-syndrome patient, the post-stroke patient, or the patient who has experienced head trauma. Using the developmental approach, this level parallels that of the young child who has less need of the stroking and caressing gestures of which we spoke earlier and who is now being "talked to" by the parenting figure. Speech is used as a means of orienting the child to the world and of familiarizing the child in a total way with the environment.

Similarly, the geriatric patient, due to both organic processes and environmental changes, has been given less attention and may therefore have lost his or her former reality-based orientation to the world. When the structure of the environment is not communicated often and in a continuous way, as is frequently the case in institutions, there may be no need to know that Monday is Monday and that it is different from Saturday. Our real world consists, not only of abstract knowledge of the world, but also of structures within each day that bring home the fact that, for example, Monday is a workday, and Sunday is part of a nonwork weekend. When the geriatric patient is in an environment in which one day leads into another and in which there are no boundaries or structures to define what it is that makes up that day, there can be a sense of loss of "day-ness," "time-ness," or "place-ness." It is this patient who is best suited for reality-orientation therapy.

As with the patient assigned to sensory training, the best way to determine if he or she is suited to reality orientation is to talk with the patient. The worker can ask for simple information, such as: What day is it today? What is the weather like? What holiday is coming? If there is difficulty in most of these areas, the worker can assume that the patient is suited to reality-orientation therapy.

Sometimes it is difficult to determine if the patient should be assigned a lower-level technique, such as sensory training, or a slightly higher one, such as reality orientation. The best way to determine this is to assess which of the behaviors mentioned earlier are most characteristic. Does the patient seem so withdrawn that sensory awakening would be helpful, or does he or she seem to have no problem in this area but to have difficulties in orientation? Again, although the patient may show signs of needing both therapies, it is best to assign the treatment modality needed *most* at the time of assignment.

Since these techniques are arranged hierarchically (i.e., sensory training is on the lower level, with the others ranked above it), it is best, when in doubt, to first assign the patient a lower-level technique. This stepladder approach prevents insulting the patient's sense of self. Rather than being assigned a higher-level technique and then being "demoted," the patient is assigned a lower-level therapy with the possibility that the worker underestimated his or her functional level and can then reassign or promote the patient to a higher-level technique.

A reliable and valid scale for measuring the degree of overall functioning in geriatric patients is the *geriatric rating scale*.[2] This is easy to administer, because it can be done on the wards by staff personnel and requires no special training on the part of the rater. In addition, the patient need not be cooperative or even present during the rating (see Appendix A). This scale has been found helpful in ascertaining the characteristics of geriatric patients before they participate in the programs that we have described.

The Least Regressed Patient: The Third Step

Remotivation therapy follows reality orientation. Using our developmental model, we may use the analogy of the young child who is now in a classroom setting. Having been stroked and talked to by parenting figures, the child is now in a structured environment in which he or she is learning about the real world. Similarly, the geriatric patient is in need of a structured group setting in which an intellectual interest in the world is restimulated. As with sensory training and reality orientation, the worker can best assess which technique is most suited to the patient by talking with the patient and with other staff. The geriatric rating scale mentioned earlier may also be helpful.

Remotivation therapy is a structured technique that includes definite steps. In many ways, it is similar to a classroom experience with a teacher (the worker) and with students (the geriatric patients). The worker uses a prepared folder similar to a class lesson plan. The exercise asks for concrete information of a "school" nature. Topics include stamps, holidays, travel, fashions, and others. Focus is on the accuracy of the response. In addition, whereas, in sensory-training and reality-orientation therapies, individual attention is given to each patient, here the focus, though individual, is on the group. Patients are not stroked and touched, as in the preceding techniques. The patient chosen for this technique is one who is regarded as functioning on a higher level than those in either of the two preceding groups.

REFERENCE NOTES

1. Drummond, L., Kirchhoff, L., & Scarbrough, D. R. A practical guide to reality orientation: A treatment approach for confusion and disorientation. *The Gerontologist*, December, 1978.
2. Plutchik, R., Conte, H., Lieberman, M., & Weiner, M. B. Reliability and validity of a scale for assessing the functioning of geriatric patients. *Journal of the American Geriatrics Society*, 1970, *18*, 491–499.

6

Sensory Training

BACKGROUND AND GOALS

Sensory training is used effectively with the regressed older person who shows an inability to interact with his or her environment. The goal is to literally bring this individual back in touch with the surroundings. A structured group–individual experience that involves all five senses, its aim is to provide the older person with differentiated stimuli to improve perception of, and response to, the physical and human environments. This technique, developed in 1968 by Leona Richman when she was Director of Occupational Therapy at the Bronx Psychiatric Center, is geared to the more regressed institutionalized geriatric patient who formerly had little opportunity for activity or group participation with trained staff.

At one time, the more regressed patient in a rehabilitative setting had little or no treatment modalities available, although better-functioning patients could take advantage of occupational therapy, recreational therapy, activities of daily living, psychotherapy, and other modalities. These activities required a long attention span, small- and large-muscle control, perceptual motor coordination, socialization skills, and the ability to follow instructions. Only the more able, self-motivated patients, therefore, could take advantage of the available rehabilitative activities.

Sensory training attempts to combat the effects of physical, social, and psychological breakdown in the more regressed geriatric patient by either maintaining the patient's present level or by avoiding further decompensation. The bodily contact and social interaction that this approach involves has also been known to alleviate depression.[1]

Sensory training breaks the environment into its most simplified and comprehensible form. Simple body-awareness exercises and sensory stimuli are presented, experienced, reacted to, and understood by the patients. The environment then becomes predictable and "deconfused." The peers with whom the patient is interacting, along with the leader, provide an opportunity for interaction, for recognition by others and, most essentially, for feedback on behavior that may then be amenable to change.

THE TARGET POPULATION

Patients appropriate for this technique exhibit deficiencies in any or all of the following areas: perceptual motor ability, sensory input discrimination, and psychosocial performance. The regressed patient who is socially withdrawn, for example, would benefit from sensory training. Verbal proficiency is not necessary, and patients who lack the use of one of the senses (such as the blind or the deaf) should not be excluded from the group, because the training experience will help them to learn to use other senses more efficiently and to compensate for the sensory loss.

COMPOSITION OF THE GROUP

Ideally, there should be between five and seven patients in a group and a balance of verbal and nonverbal members. A group may function well, however, with as few as four members or as many as ten.

Groups should consist of members who are at the same functioning level. In order to determine which patients are best suited for this technique, there should be consultations with staff members who are most in contact with the particular patient on a daily basis. It must be determined whether or not the patient is having difficulty interacting with the environment primarily because of a sensory loss. Several staff members should agree that a particular patient would benefit most from sensory training at this particular time.

Not all patients have to be at the same level of regression. It is often helpful to have a ''sparker'' in the group; that is, a member who, by virtue of a higher level of participation, enthusiasm, interest, and rapport with the leader, can help keep the group lively. This patient can also function as a model for the others to imitate.

TIME

Experienced staff have suggested that the best time for sensory training is in the morning, when patients are generally well rested and more alert. The day may be started with sensory awakening and awareness as preparation for the rest of the day. The group session may last approximately one hour, although initial sessions may be shorter because of the patients' short attention span and unfamiliarity with the group experience. Later, as the group becomes more cohesive, and as the members become more comfortable with one another and with the experience, the session may last longer. Time of day, however, may have to be modified to best suit the needs of the patients, the staff, and the institutional schedules. If the physical therapist comes only in the morning and if some members of the group receive physical therapy, morning would not be the appropriate time. If patients try to leave the group during the first few sessions because they become restless, it may be helpful to shorten the session. A shorter session is better than no session at all, and shorter sessions at more frequent intervals are still better.

FREQUENCY

The greatest progress will be seen if the session is conducted every day, seven days a week. If this is not feasible, five times a week would also be very beneficial. In some facilities, however, there are as few as two sessions per week. The number of times weekly, like the time afforded each session, will be determined according to the support of the administration, other duties of the leader, other activities offered to this patient group and, in general, the total schedule of the institution. Total familiarity with the institution's activities (including meal times, bath times, religious services, and visiting) is necessary in order for the leader to choose a time that does not conflict with other programs.

PLACE

The group should meet in the same place every time. The room should be quiet, comfortable, and well lit. It should be out of the way of mainstream activity so that the group is not distracted by other patients or staff. It should be a room that group members can think of as *their* meeting place. The room should not be too large or cluttered, and the atmosphere should be one of intimacy. Chairs should be arranged in a circle to allow for the highest level of interaction among members and to permit them to observe each other. This affords the greatest involvement in a total sharing experience that is both verbal and nonverbal. Chairs should have enough room between them so that the group leader feels free to move between them but should not be so distant that the closeness of the group situation is lost. Patients in wheelchairs should be included in the circle, and there should be enough space between wheelchairs to allow the leader to move around between them.

MATERIALS

No special materials are needed for sensory-training exercises. Simple, everyday objects will do for the sensory-stimulation portion. For the sense of smell, one could bring in a freshly cut flower, some tobacco, or some perfume. To stimulate hearing, one could bounce a ball, clap hands, or ring a bell. For touch, one could use sandpaper, a piece of velvet, a steel-wool soap pad, or a piece of cotton. For vision, one could use a hand mirror or a set of differently colored and/or shaped objects. For taste, the options are wide. One could reinforce the sessions by offering goodies or refreshments at the close.

The major point here is that nothing special has to be purchased. What is readily available in the facility is all that is needed. The primary factor is the leader's interest and creativity.

A WRITTEN SCHEDULE FOR REINFORCEMENT

It has been found most useful to have the sensory-training group schedule—time, day, and place—plus the names of the participants posted in conspicuous places on the ward. This reminds staff, patients, the administration, visitors, and all others that sensory training is being conducted or that "something is happening on the wards." It also helps patients to remember where they are to go, at what time, and on what day. It reinforces memory because it activates memory traces that could otherwise become atrophied through disuse.

It has been found most helpful to have these listings displayed in several places along the ward, such as near the day room, outside the nurses' quarters, and outside the area where the sensory training session is being held. The best way to exhibit this information is to write it in large block letters in dark ink to ensure maximum visibility.

THE LEADER

The leader, or the one trained in the sensory-training technique, may be a staff member, a volunteer, or even another patient. Sensory-training sessions are conducted by people from a variety of disciplines, such as nursing, occupational therapy, recreational therapy, physical therapy, social work, and psychology. Volunteers may also learn and apply this technique. In addition, it has been found that more intact patients can sometimes learn this approach and can be used as ancillary therapists. In other words, any person who is motivated and believes that the regressed geriatric patient can be helped by therapeutic approaches may learn and apply this technique successfully. The leader of a particular group should remain with that group as consistently as possible. Since there may be several sensory-training groups conducted throughout a given facility by a variety of staff, these leaders should exchange information and experiences regularly in order to better understand how their patients are progressing.

ROLE OF THE LEADER DURING A SESSION

The leader is responsible for establishing a friendly, nonthreatening atmosphere. Group members should find each session a comfortable, positive, and rewarding experience. The leader accomplishes this by accepting patients as they are and by emphasizing their abilities and contributions through reinforcing correct responses and ignoring incorrect responses. Eye contact is used as much as possible. The group leader may have to squat at the side of the patient with whom he or she is working in order to establish and maintain eye contact when speaking. The leader who has a "warm" quality and who can comfortably touch a patient has been found to be successful with those in sensory training.

It should be emphasized that sensory training is *not* primarily a classroom or teaching situation and that correctness of response is not the prime factor. What is important is the patient's experience within the total context of the group situation. Different members of the group may perceive the same stimulus in various ways. The leader is not to correct the participant because he or she gives the "wrong" answer. Instead, each member's perceptions are to be accepted and appreciated. In this way, the patient feels free to offer responses and obtains reinforcement with each response. This encourages self-confidence and self-esteem, essential components of the total group experience.

SENSORY-TRAINING TECHNIQUE

Orientation

The leader greets each group member by name and introduces each member to the rest of the group. Although first names usually help to establish an informal atmosphere, the leader should be sensitive to the patient's feelings about this and should use surnames whenever a patient seems to need this kind of courtesy. It has sometimes been helpful for the leader to say something like "Shall I call you Mrs. C. or Sara? Which do you prefer?" The leader must sensitively use his or her own judgment. Name tags are helpful for both patients and leader. Names should be written in large letters so that they can be read easily. Both the patient's first and second names should appear on the tag.

The leader should comment on something that each member is wearing or on the consistency of attendance at the meetings, because these comments make each person feel welcome and reinforce positive behavior. Remarks such as "Mrs. G., you look so nice with your hair combed that way," or "Mr. S., it is so good to see you coming to all of these sessions" have proven helpful.

Once greetings have been concluded, the group should be oriented to the time and place. For example, the leader may say, "Today is Monday, June 5th, and we are meeting in the day room of XYZ Place." The leader then tells the group the purpose of the meeting—that they are there to do exercises and that they will be doing two kinds of exercises, for the body and for the mind. The leader then outlines the benefits of doing the exercises and why it is important for everyone to do them. This may include information such as "These exercises help us identify our body parts," or, "Our exercises for our mind help us remember, and that makes us feel good." Having been introduced and oriented as to time, place, and purpose, the group is ready to begin the next segment of the session.

Body-Awareness Exercises

During the second portion of the session, the different body joints are identified. The leader may say, "We are now going to exercise our wrists. Here is my wrist, and this is how it moves." The major purpose of this is to give patients a sense of body awareness and to explain the obvious benefits of moving body parts that might ordinarily remain motionless. It is considered more important for patients to be able to identify their body parts than to do the actual exercises. Whenever possible, each member of the group should do each exercise.

Specifically, the joints on the arm to be exercised are the shoulders, elbows, wrists, and fingers. The legs are exercised by moving the knees and the ankles. The neck and the waist might also be exercised. It is important for the leader to follow a structured sequence when introducing each joint. He or she should progress from the top of the body (shoulders) to the bottom (ankles). There is then a review in which the leader verbalizes what has just been done, such as, "We have just finished exercising our wrists."

Stimulation of the Senses

The third segment involves *sensory stimulation*. In this phase, the five senses and their corresponding sensory organs are identified. These senses are stimulated by a variety of props (a flower, a cookie, a mirror brought in by the leader or found in the room) and are reacted to by the group members. It is essential that each sense be stimulated in each session and that each group member has an opportunity to respond to each stimulus.

The leader should start with sight and end with taste. The group members are told that they will exercise the sense of sight by using their eyes. The leader identifies her or his own eyes and helps the group members find theirs. The group may then be presented with something to see (a mirror) and asked to respond to, not identify, what they see. Questions such as "Do you like what you see?" or "How do you look today?" may be asked. The leader then repeats to the entire group what the individual group member said, such as "Sara said she looks nice today" or "Mr. J. says he sees his own face." Not only does this stimulate sight, but it also heightens self-awareness.

Taste may be left for last, since the stimulus serves as a reward—a sucking candy or cookie for those whose diets permit this (other foods are used for those whose diets do not permit sweets). Group members usually enjoy this very much.

The leader encourages appropriate responses by phrasing questions in accord with each person's level of functioning. Better-functioning patients may be able to answer a question such as "How does this smell?" when presented with the odor of tobacco or perfume. This question might be difficult for a more withdrawn patient to answer. The leader might ask this patient, "Can you smell this?" or "Do you like this smell?" These questions require little cognitive ability, such as the simple identification of the presence of an odor, and allow a nonverbal patient the opportunity to respond. When the patient does respond to a presented stimulus (for example, the sound of a ball being bounced by the leader), the leader repeats the patient's verbal response to the entire group. When the response is nonverbal (such as a nodding of the head indicating "yes" to the question "Do you like this smell?"), this response is also interpreted for all to share. The leader may nod her head and say, "Sara is nodding her head because she likes this smell."

Conclusion

In the final segment of the session the leader asks the group members for feedback on their enjoyment of the session and may repeat some of the members' comments. Before concluding the session, the leader announces the time and place for the next meeting and thanks each member for coming. He or she may use a personal greeting for each group member, along with general comments, such as "Thank you for coming. I hope that you enjoyed it. See you next (day) at (time) o'clock at (place)."

Immediately after the session's conclusion, the group leader should complete a written evaluation of what has happened while it is still fresh in her or his mind (see Appendix B). It is most essential that the evaluation be made *before* the leader's memory fades. This also ensures documentation of progress over time. Documentation makes it easier for the staff to understand how the group experience has affected the functioning level of a particular patient. It is direct evidence of a line of growth that has to be charted in order to be fully understood. Such documentation also serves as a record to be used for determining if the patient should continue at this level or perhaps be promoted to the next. Record keeping is most essential, whether the leader uses the evaluation forms provided in this appendix or makes up his or her own.

PRIMARY AND SECONDARY LEVELS OF SENSORY TRAINING

There are two levels of sensory training: primary and secondary. The primary level is used for the more regressed and withdrawn patients. It is concrete and extremely structured, and the tasks are simple. Using this level, the leader *tells* the group members everything instead of asking them questions. There is one simple exercise for each body part, usually involving an "in-out" or "up-down" motion, and there is one concrete stimulus for each sense. The leader uses a stimulus that the participants find easy to respond to; for example, a loud noise (the banging of a hammer), a harsh smell (ammonia), or a rough texture (a brush). Patients at this level are asked only if they can experience the stimulus ("Can you smell this?") and if they like what they are experiencing ("Do you like the smell?").

At the second level, called secondary sensory training, the leader adheres to the same basic structure but makes the tasks more challenging, telling the group less and asking more in order to encourage greater participation, because these group members are better able to participate. The leader might ask, "Why is it important for us to do these exercises?" She or he might introduce two exercises for each body part or might even ask group members to suggest some exercises to do. The leader could present two sensory stimuli for each sense and could ask a patient to compare the two. Wording, too, may be different. For example, the leader may introduce an adjective into the question by asking the group member to choose the adjective that he or she prefers: "Does it smell weak or strong?" "Does it feel rough or smooth?" As suggested previously, the leader repeats the group member's answer so that all members of the group will be aware of the particular response.

Primary Sensory-Training Session

The following is an example of how a leader might conduct a primary sensory-training session:

Leader: Good morning, everyone. Today, we are going to do some exercises. But first, let us introduce ourselves. My name is ______________.
[*To first group member.*]
Would you please tell us your name?
[*Leader stands just to the side of the patient so that others can see.*]

Patient: My name is Joseph.

Leader: This is Joseph. I am glad that you could join us today, Joseph.
[*To next group member.*]
Would you like to tell us your name, please?
[*Responds to second group member and continues around the circle.*]

Leader: I said that today we are here to do exercises. We are going to do two kinds of exercises—exercises for our bodies and exercises for our minds. First we will exercise our bodies, and then we will exercise our minds. Exercising makes us feel healthy and keeps us limber. We are going to exercise the parts of the body that move, called the joints. The first part that we will exercise is the shoulders.
[*Touches shoulders.*]
These are my shoulders. Can you find your shoulders?
Joseph, these are your shoulders.
[*Touches Joseph's shoulders.*]
Good, Mary is now showing us where her shoulders are. John has found his shoulders. Betty, here are your shoulders.
[*Touches Betty's shoulders.*]
Now that we have all found our shoulders, we will exercise them. We will exercise our shoulders by moving our arms up and down.
[*Raises arms up over head and then lowers them down to side. Moves around the circle, helping those having difficulty and offering both verbal and tactile praise.*]
Good. Now that we have exercised our shoulders, we will exercise our elbows. These are my elbows. Can you find your elbows?
[*Repeats as with shoulders.*]

This process is repeated, and similar wording is used for all of the joints, from the shoulders down to the ankles. Modifications may be used by the group leader, depending on his or her awareness of the needs of this particular group.

Leader: We have just finished exercising our ankles, and that completes our body exercises. We exercised our shoulders, elbows, wrists, fingers, knees, and ankles.
[*As the leader reviews these joints, she or he moves around the circle, touching one member's shoulder, another's elbow, etc., for demonstration purposes.*]
How do you feel after having done these exercises?
[*Typical responses are "tired," "O.K.," "Good," etc.*]
Now we are going to exercise our minds. It is important to exercise our minds

because we think with our minds and because our minds tell us a lot about the world around us. We will exercise our minds by using our five senses. The five senses are seeing—with our eyes; hearing—with our ears; smelling—with our noses; touching—with our fingers; and tasting—with our tongues.
[*Again, the leader lists the sensory organs, moving around the circle, touching one person's eyes, another's nose, etc.*]
The first sense that we will use is seeing, and we see with our eyes.
[*Points to own eyes.*]
Can everyone find their eyes?
[*Leader helps those who have difficulty finding their eyes and offers praise for all as they point to their eyes.*]
Now I have something here that we are going to see with our eyes. This is a mirror, and we use a mirror to see ourselves. Joseph, I'd like you to look in the mirror, please. Can you see yourself?
[*Leader kneels to the side of the patient and holds the mirror so that Joseph can see his reflection, if Joseph cannot hold the mirror himself. If the patient can hold the mirror, he is encouraged to do so.*]
How do you look today?
[*Leader repeats the response to the group.*]
Mary, can you see yourself in the mirror?
[*Each patient then gets an opportunity to look in the mirror and to respond to this stimulus.*]
Now that we have used our eyes to see, we are going to use our noses to smell. This is my nose. Where is your nose?
[*Again, the leader helps those who have difficulty locating their noses and offers both tactile and verbal praise to all.*]
I have something here that I'd like you to smell. Tell me if you like it.
[*Leader holds stimulus so that everyone can see it and so that no one is taken by surprise.*]
Mary, I have something here for you to smell. Can you smell it?
[*Waits for response.*]
Do you like the smell?
[*The responses to both this and the preceding question are repeated to the group. Each member gets a chance to respond to the stimulus. Responses are always repeated for the group.*]
So far, we have exercised our eyes to see and our noses to smell. Now we will use our ears to hear.
[*Members are asked to locate this sensory organ.*]
I have a mallet, and I am going to make a noise with it.
[*Leader bangs once sharply.*]
Did everyone hear that? Now I am going to make that noise a number of times, and I'd like everyone to listen with their ears; try to count the number of times you hear it.
[*Leader bangs distinctly from two to five times and asks each member how many times he or she heard the noise. If one patient says that he or she heard a different number of bangings from another patient, the difference is not noted. What is important is that each patient did hear the noise.*]
We have exercised our senses of seeing, smelling, and hearing. Now we will exercise our sense of touch by using our fingers. These are my fingers. Show

me yours. I have a brush. I am going to rub you across your fingers with this brush.
[*Holds the brush so that all can see.*]
I would like you to tell me if you like the way the brush feels. Joseph, I am going to rub you with the brush.
[*Holds the patient's hand palm up and lightly rubs the patient's fingers with the brush.*]
Can you feel this? Do you like the way it feels?
[*Repeats response to the group.*]
The last sense that we will exercise is the sense of taste. To taste, we use our tongues. This is my tongue. Where is yours? I have something that I would like you all to taste.
[*Leader passes out a stimulus to all patients and then asks for individual responses.*]
Mary, can you taste the candy? How does it taste to you?
[*Responses are repeated for the group.*]
Well, today we have done a lot of exercises. We exercised our bodies, and we exercised our minds by using our five senses. Did you enjoy doing these exercises? Shall we do them again? We will do them again tomorrow morning at ten o'clock. Thank you all for coming.
[*Leader shakes each member's hand, thanks each one for coming, and makes an appropriate and rewarding personal comment to each member of the group.*]

Secondary Sensory-Training Session

The following is an example of how a leader might conduct a beginning secondary sensory-training session.

Leader: Good morning, everyone. Today we are going to do some exercises. But first, let us introduce ourselves. Does anyone remember my name?
[*Stands behind a patient's chair.*]
Now, does anyone remember this lady's name?
[*Stands behind another patient's chair.*]
Now, what is this man's name? Good.
[*Leader says "good" if the patient is correct; if the patient is wrong, the leader does not allude to the mistake but goes on to ask another patient. If this, too, proves unsuccessful, the leader then states the person's name.*]
Does anyone know what today's date is?
[*Uses this technique until the correct response is obtained from a group member; if this does not happen within a reasonable time, the leader gives the correct answer.*]
What is the name of this place that we are all in?
[*Again, uses the technique described for giving person's name and date.*]
We are going to do two kinds of exercise today. First, we will exercise our bodies, and then we will exercise our minds. Is it important to exercise our bodies? Why is it so important?
[*Gets a response from one of the members.*]
Good. We will exercise the parts of our bodies that move, called the joints. Can anyone remember the first part of our body that we exercised? Yes, it is

the shoulders. Can anyone show us how we exercise the shoulders?
[*Waits for response.*]
Good.
Now that we have exercised our bodies, we will exercise our minds. Why is it important to exercise our minds?
[*Waits for appropriate response from a group member.*]
Good. We will exercise our minds by using the five senses. Does anyone remember any of the five senses?
[*Waits for response and reinforces an appropriate one.*]
The first sense that we will exercise is the sense of sight. What do we use to help us see? We use our eyes. John, how many people do you see in this room? Is anyone wearing red clothing? Is anyone in this room wearing blue clothing?
[*Again, reinforces appropriate response.*]
Can anyone see anything in the room that has a square shape? A round shape?

Other examples of vision exercises that may be used are (1) "Simon Says," (2) describing the appearance of others in the group and their clothing, (3) describing the colors, furnishings, and decorations (such as paintings) in the room.

Leader: Now we will exercise the sense of hearing. What do we use to hear with? Am I speaking in a loud voice or in a soft voice? Mary, say "hello" to Pat in a loud voice. Now Pat, say "hello" to Mary in a soft voice.
[*Technique continues as before, repeating each response and reinforcing it.*]
I'd like everyone to close their eyes and try to identify the noise that I make.
[*Noises to be made may be in the form of keys rattling, paper crumpling, door slamming, hands clapping, or whistling.*]
I'd like everyone to close their eyes. I am going to make a loud noise, and I would like everyone to listen and tell me from which part of the room the noise is coming. Now we will exercise our sense of smell. What do we use to smell with? What are some of the things that smell good to you? What are some of the things that smell bad to you?
I have two things here that I would like you to smell.
[*Has perfume and turpentine.*]
Which smell do you like better? Which is stronger? Can you identify them?
The next sense that we will exercise is the sense of touching. What do we use to touch with? John, can you touch Mary's hands? Do they feel warm or cold? Mary, how do John's hands feel?
[*Holds Mary's hand.*]
Whose hand is warmer, John's or mine?
I have two objects here that I would like you to feel.
[*Rubs patient with sandpaper and silk.*]
Roberta, which is smoother?
I have a bag here filled with different objects (pencil, ball, cup, toothbrush, safety pin, button). I'd like you to reach into the bag, grab an object and, with your eyes closed, try to identify the object just by touching it.
[*As always, appropriate responses are reinforced and repeated to the group.*]
The last sense that we will exercise today is the sense of taste. What do we use to taste with? I have two things here (a cracker and a sourball candy) that I would like you to taste.

[*Hands each one a cracker.*]
What kind of a taste does that have?
[*Hands each one a sourball after making sure that this and the cracker are allowed on everyone's diet.*]
What kind of taste does that have? Which taste did you like better?
[*In addition, the leader might have the patients identify different flavors in a pack of candies.*]
Those are the exercises for today. How did you enjoy these exercises? Shall we do them again? We will do them again tomorrow morning at ten o'clock. Thank you all for coming.
[*Shakes each patient's hand and again offers each one a personal statement.*]

INNOVATIONS IN TECHNIQUE: USING ASSOCIATIONS

It has been found helpful to use associations in secondary-level sensory-training sessions. For example, after a patient has been stroked with a brush, he or she may be asked, "What does it remind you of?" Similarly, after being stroked with velvet, a patient might say that it feels "soft" or "cuddly." One who has been encouraged to associate might say, "Like a dress I used to have. I wore it at a wedding a long time ago." The leader may then go on to stimulate other memories, such as when the wedding took place, whose wedding it was, the color of the dress, the meaning of the event to the patient. This modification allows the patient to reminisce, providing additional meaning to the sensory-training experience and reactivating the memory traces of former life, linking past and present. Association provides an additional integrative function for the patient.

The leader should use associations to heighten the experience of group members, trying to give each one an opportunity to associate and reinforcing each response with comments like "It sounds like you really enjoyed wearing that velvet dress, Mrs. G. You must have looked lovely."

Using associations as an ancillary technique also provides the leader with additional information about the patient's life that can be filed away and used at other times, such as when sitting and chatting with the patient. The leader may also share this information with other staff members, because these additional facts may be of help in planning activities and in understanding choices of friends and general current behavior.

LEADERSHIP TECHNIQUES

Every group leader eventually develops his or her own style, but a new leader needs guidelines. The following suggestions may be helpful.

Use Repetition

Repetition is an essential part of the total group process and of group interaction. Nonverbal repetition is valuable to those who are hard of hearing or whose attention spans are short. Repeating verbal responses permits everyone to share the responses, gives feedback to the contributing group member, and acts as a reinforcer for the entire group. If a response is repeated often, it is likely to appear over and over again.

Call the Patient by Name

The patient's name should be used frequently. This gives recognition to the person, and verbalizing reinforces both the group and the contributing member to remember the name. All appropriate verbal and nonverbal responses should be repeated by the leader. Inappropriate responses should be deemphasized by not repeating them.

Structure the Session

Patients should be encouraged to strictly follow the structure of the session. Digressions hinder concentration and lessen the cohesive structure of the group. Comments that do not pertain to the sequence of the session can be dealt with at the end of the session by the leader, who may state that fact in a cursory, though receptive, way.

Move Around

The leader should be in constant motion and should never stand in any one place too long, because this decreases the impression that the leader is the dominant teacher. The leader should move around to each patient as he or she responds and should stand next to or behind the patient's chair. This prevents the rest of the members from being excluded. Thus, the group is not dominated by just one person, the leader.

Touch the Patient

Touching is a very essential part of this particular technique. It conveys a feeling of warmth and acceptance to the other person. It says, in effect, "I am here, and I care." Touch is a form of communication and reward. As the leader moves around the group, therefore, he or she should touch each patient on the shoulder or arm in order to create a warm, accepting atmosphere. When the individual patient responds to the stimulus presented, the leader should touch him or her and should repeat the response that the patient has just offered. This helps the other patients to focus on who is responding and serves as a reward that is easily understood by the responding group member.

Praise the Patient

The leader uses praise as a reward. Each response is recognized by the leader with a comment such as "good," "fine," "very nice," or a similar form of verbal recognition. In addition, eye contact should be maintained at all times in order to encourage additional responses and to further create a feeling of warmth between the leader and each patient.

Adjust the Tempo of the Session

The leader's voice should be loud and clear, and he or she should *speak slowly*, projecting the voice so that everyone in the group can hear. The tempo of the session should be slow and smooth. When the leader appears to rush through the session, the group may have the impression that the leader wants to get it over with quickly. Older people are slower in responding to stimuli, in processing "input." If one of the goals in this technique is to "deconfuse" the environment, rushing through the session may mean that some group members are going to miss some aspects of the group experience.

The leader should also allow ample time for each group member to respond. The total process of receiving sensory stimulation, understanding or integrating it, and reacting to it in the form of an expressed response takes varying amounts of time. The group member who takes a little longer than others to respond should not be penalized. The leader should understand and should work *with* the differences in response time.

QUESTIONS AND ANSWERS ABOUT SENSORY TRAINING

How Can a Disruptive Member Be Handled? In a primary group, it is very important not to have any disruptions. If a member is disruptive, the leader should indicate that members can stay in the group only if they can control their behavior but that, if they cannot, they will be asked to leave. Sometimes this is enough for change to take place. If the patient refuses to be quiet, however, he or she should be firmly (but kindly) escorted out of the session and told that perhaps the next time they will be able to join the group and stay for the whole session. This can be tried for two or three sessions but, if there is no improvement, the patient should be dropped from the group. The group must not be sacrificed for the individual.

In a secondary group, in which the members are more aware and more verbal, the leader should ask the other patients what they think of the disruptive member's behavior, thus eliciting peer-group pressure if it is needed. Group members will usually say that they find some actions distracting and that the disruptive member should be quiet and listen. Often, patients will yield to this peer-group pressure, but if they do not, they should be asked to leave but should be given the option to return if their behavior improves. This gives patients a sense of mastery and choice over their behavior.

If the leader considers the disruptive member capable, he or she could ask the member to act as a co-leader. By leading one of the exercises or by helping a less capable member, the disruptive patient receives, in a more positive and constructive way, the attention that he or she craves.

What About People Who Do Not Like to Be Touched? To most people, touching conveys a feeling of warmth and closeness and is usually appreciated. Occasionally, however, there will be a patient who does not want to be touched. The leader should accept this. A feeling of closeness can be obtained in other ways, and the patient should not be ignored. The leader should stand near the person during the session, perhaps touching the back of the person's chair. Shaking hands and doing exercises in pairs are more acceptable forms of touching for some people. Gradually, as the group experience progresses, the patient may begin to see touching as a nonthreatening form of communication and may even welcome it.

How Are Handicapped Patients Integrated into the Group? When a handicapped patient (for example, one who is blind) is introduced into the group, the leader should, at first, explain in detail what is taking place throughout the session. The blind patient is thus able to understand and follow the process. The leader can also help the blind person with the exercises until he or she becomes familiar with the routine. When the leader begins the sensory exercises, he or she should explain to the group both the fact that the patient is blind and the ramifications of this. When the sight exercise is being performed, the other patients may look at the blind person and describe how he or she looks, what the patient is wearing, and so on. This is helpful because it enables the blind patient to obtain an image of how he or she looks and allows the patient to interact with his or her peers. The blind person may be made aware of the fact that these senses are still functioning and that they may help to compensate for the loss of sight.

Deaf and foreign-speaking patients can be dealt with in a similar fashion. Since the sensory-training session is very structured and sequential, it is easily understood. Exercises can be imitated, with the leader or other patients acting as models. Verbal responses may not be understood, but facial expressions and mannerisms can be explained by the leader or by group members.

Doesn't Repetition Become Boring? The structure of sensory training does not become boring to the patient unless he or she is on a higher level of functioning, in which case, the patient should be moved to a more demanding group, such as reality orientation or remotivation. Repetition offers the patient an opportunity to use memory, to be able to predict events, and to develop a sense of mastery, all of which is intended to improve self-confidence. If a patient becomes bored, he or she should either be given more tasks to do or be promoted.

What Is the Procedure for Moving a Patient to a Higher-Level Group? As a patient improves and is ready to graduate to a higher level, he or she should attend both groups for a few sessions and then be gradually dropped from the lower-level group. This allows the patient time to adjust to a new, more demanding group while separating from an old, mastered group.

What Is the Usual Duration of a Group? The amount of time that a group continues to meet varies greatly according to the patients, the leader, and the institution. Some patients never progress to a higher group but are able to maintain their functioning in a primary sensory-training group. At this point, it is up to the staff and the institution to determine how long the group is to function; it could function indefinitely. In some institutions, the leader works with a group for a specific period of time. If some patients are not progressing, they are dropped so that new patients may be afforded the group opportunity. In this way, those who seem to have more potential receive treatment. Sometimes, a patient may not respond for a few months or even a year but may then seem to improve. Each patient should be given ample time for change to occur. Some progress can usually be seen within two to three months.

Should Records Be Kept? Records of each session should be kept in order to enable the group leader to evaluate patients' progress over time. Each patient's responses to each session should be recorded as soon after a session as possible so that the leader will not forget any important details (see Appendix B).

Isn't This Technique Patronizing to the Aged Person? Because of its simplified structure, it is often felt that sensory training may be patronizing to the older adult. It is not a patronizing technique, however, because the tasks are realistically based on the fact that these patients are extremely regressed. Nonetheless, it is a good idea for the group leader to modify the tone and level to coincide with the patients' backgrounds and abilities. For example, a man who has been an engineer might enjoy working with shapes and forms as a means of re-identifying formerly familiar stimuli.

CHARTING PROGRESS

The best measure of progress is a well-kept record of each session (see Appendix B). By charting a patient's responses immediately after each session, the group leader develops an accurate, ongoing profile of the patient's behavior. If well-documented reports are made over a specified period, a patient's progress (or lack of it) will become evident.

If the leader uses a sensory training evaluation form, he or she circles the number of the item that corresponds most closely to the patient's response to the task described during that particular session. For example, if the patient was able to identify body parts sometimes, but not always, during that session, then "sometimes" or "1" would be the appropriate rating for that patient for that day. In addition to rating all of the responses to the different program components, ratings are also given to indicate the patient's general level of interest and enjoyment during each session. The leader might also periodically ask other staff members if there is any carry-over of behavior. When patients' behavior shows that they are ready for a more advanced group, they should be moved to one. Progress is indicated by the changes in individual item scores (there are no data available on cumulative scores). The evaluation form was developed for the purpose of noting individual changes over time. Since there are, as yet, no norms for what persons should score on this form, its importance lies in the changes that it reflects. For example, if a patient has been consistently scoring a "1" ("sometimes") on several items and suddenly begins scoring a consistent "2" ("usually"), this is a sign of progress.

The evaluation form is filled out in triplicate after each session.[2] (The state mandates a seven-day-per-week activities program, frequently recommending that the activities department be started at a rate of one-half-hour per inpatient per week.) One copy of the form is placed in the patient's medical chart (usually kept in the nursing station on each unit of each floor); one copy is kept by the group leader (to be used with his or her immediate supervisor), and one copy is sent to the chief trainer, who may be an occupational therapist, a recreational therapist, or a nurse. At the end of approximately six sessions[3] (groups may have met twice or three times a week, depending on staff duty or trained personnel available), the leader should meet with the supervisor of training to discuss each patient's progress. Both should examine the areas in which patients have made progress and those in which there has been decline. When a patient needs additional work, extra sessions should be provided. When a patient shows sufficient progress, "promotion" to a higher-level group is suggested.

REFERENCE NOTES

1. Busse, E.W., & Glazer, D.G. (Eds.). *Handbook of geriatric psychiatry*. New York: Van Nostrand Reinhold Co., 1980, p. 458.
2. Norms have not yet been established for this technique.
3. Records can be appraised after 6, 12, or 18 sessions.

7

Reality Orientation

BACKGROUND AND GOALS

Reality orientation, developed by J. C. Folsom, is an intervention strategy based on repetition and relearning that was developed for use with the moderately confused geriatric client who is disoriented as to time, place, and person. The goal is to heighten the older person's sense of reality by providing him or her with consistent, accurate information about the client and the environment. The technique was first used as an aide-centered activity program for elderly patients at the Veterans Administration Hospital in Topeka, Kansas, and went through several refinements, especially at the Veterans Administration Hospital in Tuscaloosa, Alabama.[1]

At that time, many elderly patients were placed in psychiatric facilities for lack of other available services. Such patients were relegated to the "back wards," where they received only custodial care. Here they suffered the effects of institutionalization, including depersonalization and sensory deprivation. If they were not very disoriented on admission, institutionalization often led to increased confusion. With this eventually came a nonawareness of time, place, and person.

TARGET POPULATION

In the beginning phase of rehabilitation, the reality-orientation technique adds the essential humanistic element to care of the disoriented person. Patients suffering from an organic cerebral deficit resulting from organic brain syndrome, head injuries, or stroke may benefit by this approach, as confusion may be temporary in some cases or may fluctuate from day to day.

COMPOSITION OF THE GROUP

A reality-orientation group may consist of members who exhibit a slightly wider range of function than those who are members of the sensory groups described earlier. All members may have some verbal skills, although interpersonal skills—the ability to communicate and interact with others—may vary widely.

Ideally, there should be from three to five patients in a classroom session. This number may vary, however, depending on institutional demands, such as the number of patients who could benefit from reality orientation plus the skills and training of the staff. Modification may therefore be determined by the "reality" of the institutional setting.

TIME

A time of day for reality classes depends on institutional schedules. The important factor is that classes are held at the same time every day so as to encourage a consistent environment. The following should be considered: meal schedules, shift changes, medication times, schedules of various other therapies (if the physical therapist comes in only from two to four o'clock, this would be an inopportune time for the reality class), staff availability, patient alertness, and receptivity. The class itself, however, is but one facet of the *total* reality-orientation program.

FREQUENCY

Classroom sessions should be held every day for approximately 30 minutes. If this is not possible, sessions should be as frequent as is practical, such as three times per week. It is important to understand that the classroom situation by itself is not a reality-orientation program. In fact, classroom effectiveness was found questionable when there were not also facility-wide supports and reinforcements.[2] In addition, unless the "therapists" who are instructing the classes are adequately trained and supervised on an ongoing basis, the purpose of the classroom process may become so distorted that it refutes the assumptions implicit in the technique.[3]

In a reality-orientation program, the teaching process goes on 24 hours a day on a continual basis. Information pertaining to name, time, and place can be reviewed several times each day—while the patient is grooming, at mealtimes, at the start of an occupational therapy or activities program, and so on.

PLACE

The group should meet consistently in the same place every time. The room should be comfortable, well-lit, and free of distractions. The arrangement of chairs depends on the number of participants and on the use of various props, such as a reality board, a blackboard, and other tools. Provision must be made for including wheelchairs in the seating arrangement. Ideally, patients should be seated in a circle, but this may not always be feasible. If no separate room is available, sessions can be conducted on the wards or even in a patient's room.

MATERIALS FOR REALITY ORIENTATION

Suggested materials for use throughout the facility include large, attractive clocks, calendars and bulletin boards; seasonal decorations; tray favors; and patient and staff name tags.

Possible classroom materials include individual calendars, word–letter games, blackboard, feltboard, various building-block devices for coordination and color matching, plastic numbers, large-piece puzzles, and a reality-orientation board.

Reality-Orientation Board

The reality-orientation board (Fig. 7–1) may be made by using a wooden board with slots. Words are printed on strips of cardboard, then slipped into the slots. Fixed above the slots are headings, such as the name of the institution, the year, the date (here a group member is asked the date; if the answer is correct, the date is placed on the board), the day (same as the preceding), "the next holiday is," "the weather today is" (here words such as cloudy, sunny, rainy, or windy are affixed to the board), "the last meal was" (here the meal last eaten is affixed to the board), "the next meal to be eaten" (same as in the preceding), and so on. The board can be modified depending upon the needs of the patients and the demands of the environment. Topics may range from the simple to the moderately sophisticated (Fig. 7–2).

Every session should include use of the reality board. This and similar boards should be posted on every floor because they help to orient, not only the group

NAME OF INSTITUTION	
THE YEAR IS	19__
TODAY IS	Thursday
THE DATE IS	January 14
THE NEXT MEAL IS	Supper
THE WEATHER IS	Rainy
THE NEXT HOLIDAY IS	Lincoln's Birthday

Figure 7–1. Basic setup of a reality board for classroom use. (Boards can also be used in day rooms.)

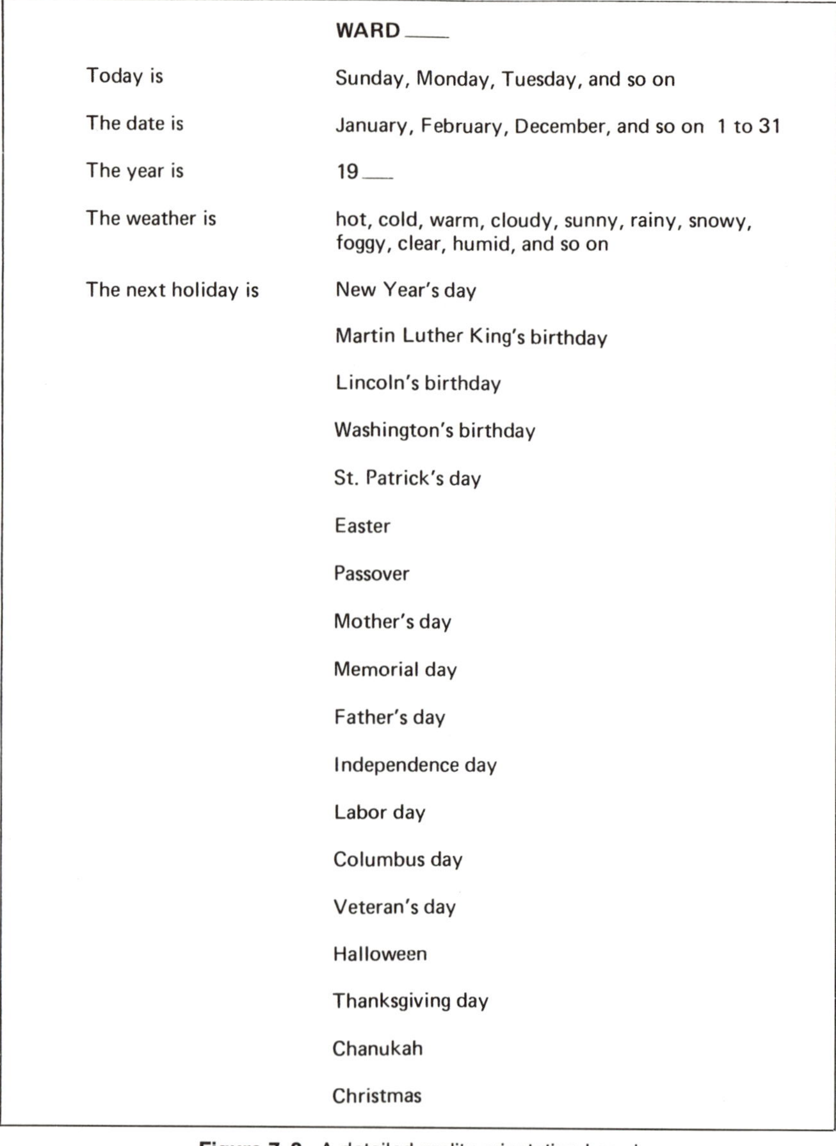

	WARD ___
Today is	Sunday, Monday, Tuesday, and so on
The date is	January, February, December, and so on 1 to 31
The year is	19___
The weather is	hot, cold, warm, cloudy, sunny, rainy, snowy, foggy, clear, humid, and so on
The next holiday is	New Year's day
	Martin Luther King's birthday
	Lincoln's birthday
	Washington's birthday
	St. Patrick's day
	Easter
	Passover
	Mother's day
	Memorial day
	Father's day
	Independence day
	Labor day
	Columbus day
	Veteran's day
	Halloween
	Thanksgiving day
	Chanukah
	Christmas

Figure 7–2. A detailed reality-orientation board.

participants, but also the general patient population. For example, in one facility, the more intact patients were observed using the board when writing letters or sending greeting cards because the board offered them needed information.

Written Schedule

It is advisable to post the schedule of sessions, as well as a list of participants, in as many conspicuous areas as possible. Perhaps the written schedule could be attached to the reality boards.

Refreshments as Reinforcers

Here is an example of how refreshments may be used as part of the program.

[*Standing in front of Mary and holding an apple.*]

Therapist: Mary, what is this?

Mary: I don't know.

Therapist: [*Hands apple to Mary.*]
What color is it?

Mary: It's red.

Therapist: That's right, Mary. It's red, and it's something to eat.

Mary: We do?

Harry: It's an apple.

Therapist: That's right, Harry. Did you hear that, Mary? It's an apple. Now, let's all taste our apples. . . .

As with sensory training, refreshments may be used as reinforcers. How and where refreshments are used (at the end of the program or as an incentive to attend) depends on the structure of the program set up by the leader. It has been found, however, that it is most useful to serve refreshments at the conclusion of a program, while the leader is informing the group about the next session.

THE LEADER

The leader should be someone who has been specially trained in the techniques of reality orientation. Although persons from different disciplines may have been trained in this area, direct-care persons (such as nursing aides) have been most actively involved in conducting reality-orientation sessions. The leader should be calm, patient, and empathic. In this technique, the leader functions more as a teacher than does the sensory-training leader. In the reality-orientation classroom, value is placed on the correctness of the patient's response, for this group is less regressed and is capable of producing correct responses. The leader must therefore encourage accurate responses and must offer reinforcement, in the form of praise, for each right answer. For example, she or he could say, "Good," "That's fine," or "You are right, Mrs. Jones."

In order to maintain an atmosphere of consistence, the leader should remain with the same group as much as possible. Provision for a consistent replacement, such as a co-leader, should be made for vacation and sick time. Whenever possible, the group should know the co-leader and should be told of the replacement in advance. This will establish and maintain a continuous tie with the leader figure. This tie has been found to be a critical factor in the success of an approach or treatment. When such a link is disrupted—when a new leader replaces the old—the functioning of the group as a whole may suffer. This disruption may cause regression of the patients, hostility toward the new group leader, a decrease in attendance, and an increase in expressed bodily ills. Once the new leader becomes the official replacement, however, and is accepted as *the* leader, these signs may vanish until the next new leader enters the scene.

Role of the Leader During the Session

The leader is responsible for establishing a warm, congenial atmosphere. She or he should therefore be accepting and empathic, and should be aware of her or his own gestures, voice, and manners and should use them for the benefit of the group. When speaking, the leader should use a strong, clear, easily understandable voice. Sentences should be short, direct, and uncomplicated in order to facilitate contact with each patient.

Although the leader should correct inaccurate responses offered by a group member, his or her manner should in no way indicate disapproval of the group member. Each person should be made to feel accepted *at all times*, regardless of the "rightness" or "wrongness" of an answer. Each member should be encouraged to offer a response but should not be made to feel guilty or ashamed when he or she does not respond properly. This unqualified acceptance of the group member by the leader helps bring about a heightened sense of self-continuity and self-esteem, the essential components and prime goals of all treatment approaches.

TWENTY-FOUR HOURS OF REALITY ORIENTATION

Reality orientation is a two-pronged program. It is conducted in the general institution, where signs, clocks, calendars, and menus identify for the patient the date, place, hour, room, meal, and activity. Above all, the individual is constantly reminded of his or her name. Bed and belongings have a name on them. The person is always addressed by name. Patients are also always reminded of the names of the persons to whom they are talking. This orientation to reality goes on during all of the patient's waking hours. Patients are continuously reminded of *who* they are, *where* they are, *why* they are here, and *what* is expected of them. In other words, a *24-hour reality orientation* is put into effect in order to maintain a total atmosphere of consistence.

In contrast, the structured reality-orientation classes are carried out in designated areas selected for convenience by staff personnel. If possible, classes meet for an intensive 30 minutes each day, as suggested earlier. If this is not possible, modifications may be made.

Reality-orientation sessions need not be as rigidly ordered as are sensory-training sessions, because the material to be covered depends very much on the patient's mastery of the information presented. At each session, the leader presents current information over and over—the patient's name, place, date, and so on. As the patient progresses, additional information is introduced (age, home town, occupation, family).

Each session begins with learning names; for example:

Leader: Good morning, Mr. Smith. I am Mrs. Jones.
[*Leader repeats own name if necessary.*]
I am Mrs. Jones.

Mr. Smith: Good morning, Mrs. Jones.

Leader: Good, Mr. Smith. Do you know the lady who is sitting next to you? [*Mr. Smith shrugs.*]

Leader: Mr. Smith, this is Mrs. Silvers. . . .

Or at another session:

Leader: Good morning, Mrs. Hall. I'm glad you could come today.

Mrs. Hall: I've got to get to work.

Leader: What work, Mrs. Hall?

Mrs. Hall: I'm a teacher.

Leader: Are you a teacher now?

Mrs. Hall: Yes.

Leader: Do you feel well enough to work now?

Mrs. Hall: No.

Leader: Mrs. Hall, you are here at Wayne Rest Nursing Home because you haven't been feeling well and aren't able to work.

Mrs. Hall: Here? Where? Who are you?

The leader should provide simple activities, such as having patients identify pictures, read the reality-orientation board, write their names, and do simple manipulative activities. Suggested classroom materials include individual calendars, word–letter games, blackboard, feltboard, mock-up clock, various building-block-type devices for coordination and color matching, plastic numbers, large-piece puzzles, and the reality-orientation board.

INNOVATIONS IN TECHNIQUE: USING ASSOCIATIONS

Some leaders have found that, in addition to using familiar objects (a bowl of fruit), making associations to the items is helpful. For example, a female patient may be identifying an apple in a bowl of fruit. She may be holding it and gently stroking it. It might be helpful to ask, "Mrs. Smith, what does the apple remind you of?" She may say, "I used to make applesauce at home." The leader could then say, "Yes, applesauce is made from apples. I'll bet you were a good cook. What else did you make?" This kind of dialogue can encourage patients to associate the current experience with some meaningful event in the past. It helps memory by reinforcing memory traces and gives additional significance to the experience that they are now sharing in the group. It is also a way for the leader and other group members to share some of the experiences in the patient's earlier life and, through them, to know the patient better. It has been found that association moves the group experience beyond the "children's play" sometimes referred to by patients. Association adds new dimensions.

In addition to using everyday objects, the leader may also introduce a mirror and ask patients to look at it and report what they see. Often, the responses to the images in the mirror are negative; for example, "I see only an old face with wrinkles," "What's to see?", or "I see someone about 30 years old." All of these responses reveal the "anguish over the stigmata of old age."[4] When a patient gives a negative response when looking in the mirror, other group members may be asked to tell how they see the person who is holding the mirror. Often, another group member's response is a positive one ("I see Mrs. Smith looking nice") and can be used to change the faulty perceptions of the one who is looking in the mirror. Additional positive responses can be elicited from the group. In this way, the viewing member is confronted with the fact that others see him or her as "an old lady with a very pretty face and smile," or "a man with nice coloring and wisdom lines in his face." This technique is used to induce the viewing member to accept old age and to correct any misconceptions of him- or herself.

Associations may be used with other events in the person's life. The group member is asked to look at paintings in the room, describe them, and relate them to paintings, drawings, or prints that the member may or may not have had at home. The paintings may help remind patients of past times, family, and other friends. Past and present are thus linked within the therapeutic process.

FAMILY INVOLVEMENT IN REALITY ORIENTATION

Family members should be included in the overall treatment plan whenever possible. This technique promotes continuity and consistence of treatment. When a patient is involved in a reality-orientation class, and when a consistent attitude is maintained by staff all day, it is harmful to have family members disrupt the reality orientation. They want to be "nice" and not "disturb mama," but this attitude encourages mama's nonreality-oriented statements. Therefore, family members should be taught not to agree with the patient's disoriented statements but to give the patient reality information at all times. For example, a client may be holding a doll in her arms and may be referring to it as a baby, pretending that it is alive and treating it like a real baby. It is helpful to suggest to the patient that the item that she is holding is a doll but that perhaps she wishes it were a real baby. It may be further suggested to her that her wish is based on her own need to have something to cuddle and hold next to herself, a need to have something that she can call exclusively her own. In this way, although reality is introduced and the patient is definitively told that the item is a doll and *not* the baby that she perceives it to be, her wishes are interpreted. This is done with warmth and empathy, and with no attempt to take the doll away from her. She is allowed to hold it, although it is always referred to realistically (i.e., the *doll* is a *doll*). The patient's family should be told how staff members handle this situation, and it should be suggested that the family do the same.

Encouraging the patient's disoriented statements is demeaning to the patient, and suggesting that "it is all right to be confused" is in contradiction to the stated goals of therapeutic programs, which attempt to provide reality for the client. When family members are encouraged to be part of the treatment, they are usually very supportive and become important members of the reality team. They should be informed of the patient's progress whenever possible so that they may share more directly in that progress.

REALITY-ORIENTATION TECHNIQUE: GENERAL POINTS FOR THE LEADER

Use Repetition

Begin each session with a review of basic information. The leader cannot over-review, since reality orientation is based upon repetition and relearning. If a patient is unable to give the desired response, the leader should give the correct answer and should ask the patient to repeat it. When patients have difficulty in verbal expression, they should be asked to write their responses or to express themselves in other ways, using anagrams, scrabble cubes, or magnetic letters on a board. The leader must be flexible and creative enough to use alternative means when the usual procedures prove inadequate.

Establish Attainable Goals

The leader should not expect too much at first from patients in reality orientation. Activities to be used in reorienting patients are simple: identification of familiar objects, picture recognition, word pictures, and the matching and repetition of simple information. These form the basis of the program. The leader must remember that the activity itself is not the only essential ingredient; the activity should lend itself to simple, friendly conversation. It is the comfortable, familiar conversation that builds self-confidence for the patient.

If patients seem aware of the basic information on the reality board, they should then be asked about such things as their home towns, families, and former occupations. The leader should be aware of the accuracy of these answers; thus, it is essential that she or he be familiar with the background and history of each patient.

Reinforce the Right Answer

The patient should be rewarded *immediately* after a correct response. The leader should say "good," "that's right," or "fine." If a patient does not give the correct response, the leader should say the correct response and should ask the patient to repeat it before moving on. Praise, small rewards (such as refreshments), and special favors should be used as incentives.

Maintain Coordination

At the inception of the reality-orientation program, a team leader should be designated. This could be the activities worker, a staff nurse, a group worker, an aide, or an orderly. The team leader must be thoroughly familiar with both staff and patients and must have the time to devote to making the program work. He or she must be responsible for maintaining an ongoing program of in-service training and evaluation of reality orientation. When there is staff turnover, the team leader must be responsible for orienting new staff and for integrating them into the team.

Outside resources can help get the program underway. The Veterans Administration Hospital at Tuscaloosa has various training programs, and state departments of health and state nursing-home associations can provide consultation and training.

In addition to the benefits that will accrue to the patients, increased staff involvement in reality orientation, as in any therapeutic process, tends to produce an increase in staff morale. Increased staff morale is one of the beneficial aspects of an environment conducive to overall patient improvement.

INTEGRATION OF REALITY ORIENTATION INTO THE INSTITUTIONAL ROUTINE

Again, it must be stressed that reality orientation is more than a classroom exercise on a time-limited basis. Instead, it is an ongoing, total thrust that must be integrated into the environment on a *24-hour basis*. The following suggestions are offered:

1. All staff should call all patients by their surnames and by their correct titles (Mr./Mrs./Miss/Ms.) unless a patient specifically requests the use of his or her first name.
2. It is extremely important that staff members *know* each patient, especially their social history (family make-up, former occupation, place of birth), so that appropriate information can be reinforced in casual contacts and conversations.
3. There should be many clocks, calendars, and bulletin boards to heighten patients' awareness of time, place, and events.
4. There should be an interesting, diversified program of activities appropriate, not only to time and place, but also in keeping with individual patient needs and interests.
5. The public address system, if available, should be used daily to remind patients of the day, time, and place. An example would be:

   Activities worker: Good morning. Today is Thursday, March 21. It's a sunny, spring-like day. This morning we are having the first meeting of our Garden Club at ten o'clock in the lounge. That's one-half hour from now—ten o'clock, in the lounge.

6. The dining room should have name cards, and patients should be encouraged to behave realistically; that is, to be considerate of others and to use appropriate utensils. An example would be:

   Aide: [*After seeing patient eating with knife.*]
   Mr. Smith, here's your fork for eating the meat and the peas and potatoes on your plate. Shall I butter the bread with the knife?

7. Appropriate meals should be served on special holidays, not only because this is a nice, pleasant gesture; it is also a reality vehicle.
8. Birthdays should be recognized individually by giving the patient a corsage, card, basket, or individual cake (this is in addition to the collective monthly birthday party). The birthday is a vehicle of reality, and it also adds a "homey" touch.
9. Clearly written, attractive activities schedules (weekly, biweekly, or monthly) should be given to each resident, because they help the patient to differentiate the days.
10. Visiting hours should be liberal, because they encourage contact with family and friends and tend to help keep patients in touch with reality. A

word of caution here, however: family members must be informed about the consistent attempt to keep patients oriented, and they must be asked to assist by not reinforcing patients' delusional, hallucinatory, or regressed material. For example, if mother says, "I want to go upstairs to the bedroom now," her daughter should not say, "Okay, mother" to appease her but, rather, "Mother, you are here at Wayne Nursing Home, and we are sitting right here in your room."

11. Good contact should be maintained with the community:
    a. Volunteers should be instructed, as are staff, regarding the infusion of reality into all facets of the nursing home.
    b. Community groups not only entertain the resident but also maintain contact with the outside world.
12. Because of the high incidence of visual impairment, color should be used to differentiate one room from another, one door from another, one hallway from another, and so on.
13. Lighting should be adequate. Lighting is extremely important in keeping people oriented. Dim lights often discourage environmental contact. Similarly, glare can be a problem; glare on hallway floors can be frightening and even disorienting.
14. The home should be cheerfully decorated at all times, and decorations should be appropriate to the season. Patients should be encouraged to keep some memorabilia, such as pictures of grandchildren and mementos of past trips or achievements, and staff should be instructed to take note of these.
15. Independence should be encouraged. Patients should be expected to dress and groom themselves as much as is practicable. If a patient does need assistance, an aide should do these things *with* the patient rather than *for* him or her. Whenever appropriate, adapted equipment should be used to maintain independence, including special utensils for hemiplegics, long-handled combs, zipper pulls, and the like.
16. Whenever practicable, more than one sense should be stimulated. In activities programs, the patient may receive input visually through written activities schedules and audially when the aide comes to the room and encourages the patient to attend.

QUESTIONS AND ANSWERS ABOUT REALITY ORIENTATION

Administratively, How Does One Go About Introducing a Reality-Orientation Therapy Program? First, there must be a commitment from the top. If this is to be a total thrust, everybody must participate—every staff member (including office and maintenance personnel), volunteers, and even family. It does not take long to discover that *attitudes are caught, not taught*. Before any commitment can be made, one has to honestly assess the facility and determine what modifications might be made to initiate or increase the reality thrust. Essentially, what is involved here is an attitudinal, not a financial, commitment.

What Is "Reality" for the Nursing-Home Patient? What difference does it make if it is Tuesday and not Friday? Nobody is going any place anyway. But Tuesday should be different from Friday! When the reality-orientation technique was originally conceived, it was for elderly mental hospital patients. Some of these patients progressed so well that they were assigned to other therapies (such as remotivation, occupational therapy, music therapy, speech therapy, physical therapy, or group therapy) and eventually were discharged into the community. But many of today's institutionalized patients are confined because there is no place in the community for them to go. So, if we restore them to a higher level of functioning, what then? This negativism has to be overcome. More emphasis must be placed on the *quality of life within the nursing home or facility*.

Does Reality-Orientation Therapy Create a "Better Patient"? If a "good" patient is a passive–dependent patient, the answer is no. Reality orientation tends to make patients more aware of themselves and their environment. The goal is to eventually involve patients in their environment and make *them responsible* for *their own behavior*. Patients are encouraged to again become as independent as possible. In one study, a Ward Behavior Inventory (WBI) was used as a premeasure and postmeasure of performance to monitor a comprehensive program of sensory stimulation in a nursing home. After the program had run for several months, the WBI showed an increase in disturbed behavior. When the authors examined what constituted "disturbed," they realized that the renewed environmental interest had fostered some aggressiveness and argumentativeness.[5] Although these behaviors might have indicated greater disturbance in a mental-hospital setting, they truly indicated a successful thrust here because the goal was, in fact, to get the patients more in touch with their environment.

Is the Classroom Situation too Kindergarten-Like? One must always remember that reality orientation is for the regressed patient. Some of the items used may well resemble materials that are used to teach children; for instance, the large mock-up clock. But many patients, in addition to their general regression, have real sensory impairments that dictate the use of special materials. If vision is poor, large numbers are essential; for the highly distractable, there must be a clear, legible number at every spot. Although care must be taken that the materials used are not juvenile, realism should be used in making the necessary adaptations to meet patient needs. Under no circumstances should the geriatric patient be infantilized. Indeed, although the structured reality classroom is a simulated formal learning experience for the regressed patient, the principle of reality orientation is one that should be practiced with all patients throughout any institution as a technique of *prevention* as well as *intervention*.

ADVANCED REALITY ORIENTATION: SETTING UP AN ADVANCED REALITY-ORIENTATION CLASS

The advanced reality-orientation class is for those who have made good progress in the basic class or for those who are initially less confused. While the procedures used are the same as in the basic class, the expectations are greater. Patients can be expected to name other people, such as the leader, family members, classmates, and other institutional staff members. Leader guidance is more limited here, since this group has a greater attention span and better powers of concentration, and can engage in discussion among themselves more extensively. Activities are creatively offered by the leader to accommodate the needs of the class. These activities may include "fill-in-the-blank" statements, such as reading or writing in the days of the month on an individual calendar. The leader may use audiovisual aids, such as flash cards and maps, for identification of items and places. As in all classes, the activities should be meaningful for each member and for the group as a whole.[6]

When patients have completed the basic classes, they should advance into the higher-level reality-orientation groups. As in basic classes, patients are expected to read and copy the reality-orientation board and the materials listed on the blackboard. In addition, they are provided with other materials to read and other projects to complete under the direction of the group leader. Here, spelling, writing, and some simple arithmetic problems may be used. Other activities could include reading and discussing current events or fill-in-the-blank quizzes. Discussions may center around any topic of interest to the group. Whenever possible, a group member should be asked to prepare a topic for simple discussion in the group. Emphasis should still be on reality orientation and, whenever appropriate, the days of the week, time, date, and name of the place should be mentioned.

The group leader should introduce her- or himself at each session and should welcome each group member by name and with a personal comment on the member's appearance, such as "How nice your hair looks today, Mrs. Smith," or "I see you have a new haircut, Mr. Armstrong."

CHARTING PROGRESS

In order to determine when the patient is ready to move on to another (more advanced) technique, it is essential to keep progress notes on each session. These records are to be attended to *immediately* after each session in order to allow for the least amount of memory loss on the part of the group leader. The record (see Appendix C) may be modified according to the patients in the group or the ingenuity or flexibility of the leader. The essential point is that some record of each patient's progress be kept in order to know if and when progress has taken place. The form is filled out in triplicate; one copy is for the medical chart (placed there at the end of a month), one is for the group leader, and one is for the group leader's supervisor.

A record should be kept for each patient for each session. Progress is indicated by consistent improvement on overall scores.[7] Although there may be progress in one area, such as verbal communication, other item scores may tend to remain the same. This is not to be taken as a sign of lack of improvement, since improvement will not necessarily be consistent for all items.

At the end of the six-week series, the leader should meet with the supervisor to discuss each patient's progress. At this point, decisions are made about promoting patients or continuing them in the same group and about providing additional supportive measures. Records should be appraised after 6, 12, or 18 sessions, depending on the decision of the leader and the realities of the environment.

ATTITUDE THERAPY: AN ADJUNCT THERAPY WITH REALITY ORIENTATION

Attitude therapy is usually used in conjunction with reality orientation. Basically, each patient's style of behavior is first identified. Then the staff decides upon and prescribes a staff style of behavior, an attitude toward this patient. The patient is treated *consistently*, with all staff members relating to him or her in the same way. The five basic attitudes involved are active friendliness, passive friendliness, matter-of-factness, kind firmness, and no demand. Each attitude is linked with a patient's behavioral type. Staff members express kind firmness toward depressed patients. No demands are placed upon destructive patients. Active friendliness is indicated for patients who are withdrawn or apathetic, passive friendliness for suspicious and paranoid patients. A matter-of-fact attitude best serves alcoholic and sociopathic patients.[8] These attitudes tend to reinforce those behaviors that are adaptive for the patient and to not reinforce those that are maladaptive. Although attitude therapy was developed as an adjunct to reality orientation, it may be used as a general approach to the patient. That is, a consistent way of relating to a patient, based on his or her habitual style of responding to the environment, is appropriate regardless of the patient's level of functioning and whether or not he or she is engaged in any specific treatment modality.

Active Friendliness

Active friendliness is used with the apathetic, withdrawn patient. The staff should seek out individuals who are withdrawn and who have little or no confidence in themselves and should attempt to counteract these patients' feelings of failure. As J. C. Folsom describes it, these patients must be "loved back to health."[9] An example follows:

> Mr. E., a man in his late 80s, sits in his room all day. The only time that he spends out of his room is to eat in the dining room, remaining there for only a few minutes at each meal. He has no confidence in himself and cannot even say if he feels good. All of his statements are laden with the words "maybe," "I guess so," "I don't really know."[10]

For this type of patient, the staff exhibits an attitude of active friendliness. After he has shaved, staff could say, "How nice you look!" or could compliment him on his choice of an article of clothing. Such constructive statements may help to rebuild his confidence and trust in himself. Once this trust has been re-established, he can begin to better communicate with others around him and to improve his overall level of functioning.

Passive Friendliness

An attitude of passive friendliness is used with the frightened, suspicious patient. Here, the worker should show interest and concern but should wait for the patient to make the first move. An active approach by staff would only tend to further alienate this person and should be avoided; friendly gestures may be misinterpreted and may increase the patient's "natural" suspiciousness. An example follows:

> A man, Mr. C., is in his early 60s and is confined to a wheelchair. He is overly suspicious of everyone. When someone walks into his room, his first reaction is: I wonder what he is doing here; what does he want?[11]

The staff approach should be one that says, "We are here to help you; we understand. If you want anything, let us know." This patient is given the opportunity to take the initiative. He should be encouraged to attend the reality-orientation class, but staff should not insist that he do so.

Matter-of-Factness

The goal here is to help the patient learn to take responsibility for his or her own behavior. Here, the staff is open but "matter-of-fact" with the individual. This attitude is best used with the highly manipulative person or with the person who shows social maladjustment. Staff members must be expressly clear that they are *not* to be manipulated and that this behavior will not be rewarded. It is hoped that, through this attitude, the patient will be able to begin a constructive life pattern. A typical situation follows:

> Mr. M., a man in his late 70s, has the marked characteristic of manipulating members of the staff for cigarettes. Because of his smoking habit, age, and physical condition, Mr. M. does not eat.[12]

Once a matter-of-fact attitude is begun and Mr. M. knows that he cannot go from one member of the staff to another to get cigarettes, he will become aware that, if he wants to enjoy his smoking, he must accept the fact that he must first eat. It has been found that this kind of person, often avoided by others because of his manipulative behavior, then becomes more socially accepted.

Kind Firmness

The depressed patient should be treated with kind firmness. The goal here is to help such patients focus away from themselves and to engage them in interaction with others. It is helpful to have these patients understand that they may express strong feelings, such as anger, appropriately. For example, if a patient is unwilling to get out of bed, it has been found helpful to insist that he or she do so.

> Mrs. G., a patient who shows depressed behavior, lies in bed and refuses to get up, toilet herself, or get dressed. The worker, upon entering the room, may say, "Mrs. G., you will have to get up and get dressed now. I will wait here for you and help you if you like. Then we will both walk down to the dining room for lunch. You must get up now."

No Demand

A no-demand approach is helpful with frightened, angry patients who are acting out fears. Such persons may even be in a panic state in which the only way they know how to act is by showing aggression toward everyone around them and even toward themselves. The goal is to remove pressure from these patients while letting them know that nobody is going to harm them. The staff should also let the patients know that they (the staff) will not respond to their anger. The only rules set down for them are:

1. They cannot leave the treatment area.
2. The staff will not permit them to harm themselves.
3. They cannot harm others.
4. They must take their medications.

Once these persons are in control, they should be given positive rewards and positive responses by staff.

QUESTIONS AND ANSWERS ABOUT ATTITUDE THERAPY

Who Prescribes the Attitude to Be Used? The appropriate attitude is selected by the reality-orientation team members, based on their knowledge of a patient and their observation of his or her behavior. It is sometimes helpful to use a consulting psychiatrist or psychologist, particularly when a patient's behavior does not seem clear to the team members; for instance, the patient is both withdrawn and suspicious or both agitated and depressed.

What Is the Essential Point of Attitude Therapy? The essential point is consistence. Each staff member should use the same approach in all interactions with the patient. The patient should then be able to understand what is expected of him or her and to respond accordingly. In some facilities, prescribed attitudes are made apparent to staff by the use of color-coded name tags. Pink may mean active friendliness and green may stand for matter-of-factness. These colors may be posted on the doors of patients' rooms, their beds, or any other obvious places.

What Are the Most Common Attitudes Used in Conjunction with Reality Orientation? The most common attitudes in the reality class are both active and passive friendliness. No matter what, the instructor must be supportive. Demands are minimal. As soon as the patient responds, she or he should be rewarded with praise. When a patient has mastered even the most simple task, the accomplishments should be made known to the entire team. Repetition, in both words and writing, is the keystone. Social interaction with other members of the class should be constantly encouraged.

Can the Prescribed Attitude Change? The prescribed attitude is subject to change depending upon changes in the patient's mode of behavior. Should a patient become ill and suddenly withdrawn and apathetic during the early recovery period, the staff would then adopt an attitude of active friendliness, even though the prescribed attitude for this patient may have been any one of the other attitudes. The patient's progress should be reviewed periodically.

Who Implements Attitude Therapy? There is no special "attitude therapist." It is suggested that every staff member practice this technique, since it cannot be emphasized too often that *consistence* is the key to patient progress.

Does Reality Orientation Combined with Attitude Therapy Really Work? Though reality orientation and attitude therapy have been widely used since their inception, there has been limited evaluation of either method's effectiveness.[13] Yet, some studies show that improvement does take place, although there are limitations both in the treatment approach and in the implementation of an ideal environment in which to test its true effectiveness.[14]

In one such study, both reality orientation and attitude therapy were used for institutionalized elderly adults (mean age, 83). Evaluations were conducted at the end of the first six months and again at the end of the study, when residents had been in the program for one year. They were compared with controls on all measures, including a Mental Status Questionnaire (MSQ) constructed for special use by that particular sample and modeled after a well-known scale (the Kahn-Goldfarb MSQ). Also measured were ratings on an Activities of Daily Living scale (ADL) and specially designed behavioral ratings.

Compared with the controls, the sample attending reality-orientation and attitude-therapy classes showed "slight, statistically significant improvement on the MSQ after six months." Though there was no favorable effect on ADL or behavioral measures, the authors suggest that advanced age, severity of disorientation, and disability may limit the effectiveness of reality-orientation. Most important, they reject the view of therapeutic "nihilsm," proponents of which seek reduced investment in psychosocial therapies for the disoriented.[15] "Nihilists" point out that "it is difficult to say how much a small change in MSQ score contributes to the general welfare of the disoriented patient," further contending that such measures serve only as vehicles "to organize attention to the disoriented, thereby guarding against unjustified custodial policies." Future studies are needed to assess the true effectiveness of reality orientation and attitude therapy. Currently they provide meaningful activity for disoriented and institutionalized patients while focusing attention on the need for further treatment approaches for this group.[16]

REFERENCE NOTES

1. Stephens, L. R., (Ed.). *Reality orientation*, rev. ed. Washington, D.C.: Hospital and Community Psychiatry Service, American Psychiatric Association, 1975.
2. Barnes, J. A. Effects of reality orientation classroom on memory loss, confusion, and disorientation in geriatric patients. *The Gerontologist*, 1974, *14*, 138–142.
3. Gubrium, J. R., and Sander, M. Multiple realities and reality orientation. *The Gerontologist*, 1975, *15*, 142–145.
4. Oberleder, M. Crisis therapy in mental breakdown of the aging. *The Geronotologist*, 1970, *10*, 111–114.
5. Loew, C. A., & Silverstone, B. M. A program of intensified stimulation and response facilitations for the senile aged. *The Gerontologist*, 1971, *11*, 341–347.

6. Drummond, L., Kirchoff, L., & Scarbrough D. R. A practical guide to reality orientation: A treatment approach for confusion and disorientation. *The Gerontologist*, December 1978.
7. Norms have not yet been established for this technique.
8. Busse, E. W., & Glazer, D. G. (Eds.). *Handbook of geriatric psychiatry*. New York: Van Nostrand Reinhold Co., 1980, p. 458.
9. Lamm, I. B., & Folsom, J. C. Attitude therapy and the team approach. *Mental Hospital*, 1965, *16*, 307–320.
10. Ibid., p. 311.
11. Ibid., p. 313.
12. Ibid., p. 317.
13. Citrin, R. S., and Dixon, D. N. Reality orientation, a milieu therapy used in an institution for the aged. *The Gerontologist*, October 17, 1977, *1*, 39–43.
14. Ibid., p. 39–43; Zepelin, H., Wolfe, C. S., & Kleinplatz, F. Evaluation of a yearlong reality orientation program. *Journal of Gerontology,* January 1981, *36*(1), 70–77.
15. Cohen, G. Comment, organic brain syndrome reality orientation for critics of clinical interventions. *The Gerontologist*, June 1978, *18*(3), 313–314.
16. Zepelin, H., Wolfe, C. S., & Kleinplatz, F. Evaluation of a yearlong reality orientation program. pp. 70–77; Wershow, H. J., Comment: reality orientation for gerontologists: Some thoughts about senility. *Gerontologist*, August 1977, *17*(4), 297–302.

8

Remotivation Technique

Remotivation is a structured program intended to reawaken the interest of apathetic patients to their immediate environment through an effort to reach the normal, healthy parts of their personalities.[1] A patient is promoted to remotivation when it has been determined by staff that he or she is ready for this therapeutic intervention. It may also happen that an alert patient who has never evidenced a need for sensory-training or reality-orientation therapy may be assigned directly to remotivation as the modality best suited to him or her.

BACKGROUND AND GOALS

Remotivation is a technique of simple, objective group interaction designed to help patients toward reality.[2] It was established more than 25 years ago by the late Dorothy Hoskins Smith of Claremont College, California, as a therapy for mentally disturbed patients and has since been found helpful for use with the more alert patients in institutions. The two therapeutic aims considered most essential are:

1. To stimulate patients into thinking about and discussing topics associated with the real world.
2. To assist patients to relate to and communicate with other people.[3]

Initially it was thought that personnel who work with this group of the aged should be professionals. It was soon found that the technique was easily learned by the direct-care workers (aides and orderlies) and that it could be appropriately conducted by them, since it was they who had the most contact with the patients. The process also allowed the direct-care workers to develop and maintain an increased sense of their own self-esteem because they were now active, contributing members of the therapeutic team.

TARGET POPULATION

Remotivation is appropriate for the patient who, although more alert than some, still needs a structured vehicle for socialization. This person is more verbal than those who are in sensory training or reality orientation and is capable of participating, to an extent, in a group discussion. The person's attention span is also slightly longer. There may be memory deficits, especially in recent memory; he or she may not remember what was eaten for breakfast yet be able to discuss topics that are familiar and of interest to the person, such as holidays, sports, fashions, and the like. This patient needs structure in the form of clear and consistent expectations and time-limited activities.

COMPOSITION OF THE GROUP

A remotivation group ideally consists of from 10 to 15 patients. A few of these patients may be more advanced than others and may serve as stimulators and "sparkers." Conversely, one or two slightly confused residents may also be included.

Some leaders prefer smaller groups. This depends on both the needs and the abilities of the group members, as well as on those of the group leader. In addition, space limitations and other reality factors should be considered.

Unlike sensory training and reality orientation, which allow for "regressed" behavior, remotivation demands a higher level of cognitive functioning and social interaction. When a patient exhibits disruptive behavior, she or he must be removed from the group until again ready for this form of therapy.

TIME

Remotivation sessions should be held once or twice a week, preferably at the same time in order to maintain consistence. A word of caution is due here: Scheduling remotivation may be difficult, since these patients are indeed capable of participating in a wide range of activities. An early-evening meeting, perhaps after dinner, may be best because other activities are not usually available then.

FREQUENCY

A remotivation program usually consists of a series of 12 such sessions. Each session requires from 30 minutes to an hour, depending on the needs of the group.

PLACE

The room in which the sessions take place should be comfortable, well-lit, and as free of distractions as possible. Furniture arrangements should allow for the inclusion of wheelchair patients. When the weather permits, it is possible to conduct remotivation sessions outdoors.

A WRITTEN SCHEDULE

Remotivation meetings should be well publicized. They should, of course, be included in a regular activities schedule. In addition, notices should be posted in conspicuous places; for example, on bulletin boards, along corridors, and in activities rooms.

THE REMOTIVATOR

Stressing the importance of the remotivator–trainer, a psychiatrist states: "Each patient has sick roles and healthy roles. The sick ones have come to dominate his life, but the healthy roles are not entirely dead. I, as a psychiatrist, deal mainly with the sick roles. You, as Remotivators, are in touch with the healthy roles."[4] The group leader, referred to as a *remotivation technician*, should be one who has attended a 30-hour course in remotivation techniques at a training center or nearby hospital, where such courses are often given. Remotivation technicians should be more formal in their total approach than leaders of the sensory-training or reality-orientation classes, because the remotivation technique was devised to simulate a classroom situation and is more didactic than the previously described approaches. It adheres to a rigid, precise format and requires advance preparation by the leader, who should feel comfortable in this formal setting. He or she should enjoy discussion, have a good general fund of information, and be able to follow the structured five steps, which will be described later.

Role of the Leader in the Session

As in a classroom situation, in which there is a teacher (the leader) and students (geriatric patients), the leader must be in control of each meeting from start to finish. In fact, it is the leader who opens and closes the meeting in a very prescribed fashion. It has been found that leaders who followed the structured order of the five steps are more successful than are those who do not. The only flexibilities allowed the leader are the length of the steps within each session and the choice of subject matter. (After several sessions have been conducted, it is sometimes helpful to have a patient choose a topic on which the group agrees and to allow the patient to conduct the session as a leader.)

MATERIALS FOR REMOTIVATION

Props for remotivation sessions are readily available; for example, jewelry, hats, shoes, clothing, flowers, pine cones, acorns, and leaves. Other props can be obtained from the dietary department (bread, cake, fruit, jellies, cooking utensils, beer, wine). Items such as decorations, quilts, and handmade articles may be borrowed from the occupational or activities therapy departments, and tools and cleaning utensils may be obtained from the maintenance department. Sometimes it is helpful to ask staff members or volunteers who travel on vacation to bring back souvenirs that can be used in the remotivation sessions. In this way, such items as Mexican hats, grass skirts, lava rock, mineral stones, gourds, wine bottles, decorated eggshells, foreign coins, and fancy menus can be collected. Interesting newspaper and magazine articles should be clipped for possible use. Libraries can be used for reference materials, as well as for films, filmstrips, and records. Props and other materials should be properly stored for periodic use and reuse.

TECHNIQUE

The remotivation technician selects topics recommended in manuals published by the American Psychiatric Association/Smith Kline and French Remotivation Project.[5] Topics selected should deal with the real world, such as the history of stamps in our country, presidents, fashions, holidays, or sports. Sensitive (controversial) topics are not usually dealt with.

The following five structured steps should be employed in each remotivation session:

Step I (3–5 min.) *Creating a climate of acceptance.* Greet each person by name, shake hands, make him or her feel welcome by telling the group that it is good to have the person there, establish a warm, congenial ambiance. Say something nice that you notice about each person.

Step II (5–10 min.) *Creating a bridge to reality.* Use "bounce" (interest-inducing) questions, gradually leading into the subject. Once the topic has been reached, an objective short poem relevant to the topic is read aloud as the remotivator moves around the circle (music, props, displays, and other visual aids may also be used). Any response is accepted by the remotivator, who repeats what was said or who may reinforce the response with "That's right," "Fine," "Good."

Step III (15–20 min.) *Sharing the world of reality.* Using the same type of questions, the leader develops the topic by asking planned, objective questions, such as "What is it?" "How big is it?" Participants are encouraged to speak to the remotivator and to each other.

Step IV (15–20 min.) *Appreciating the work of the world.* The aim here is to stimulate reminiscence and the sharing of experiences, ideas, and opinions that have past, present, and possibly future interest for participants. This is accomplished by investigating the type of work related to the topic, the value of that work, the profit associated with it, what training may be involved, and so on.

Step V (3–5 min.) *Creating a climate of appreciation.* The remotivator expresses enjoyment at having been with the group and summarizes what was said. He or she shows appreciation for any contributions made by the members and invites them to bring poems, songs, newspaper clippings, and other relevant items to the next session. The leader invites members to the next meeting and, if possible, gives the date and time of the next session.

The following is a transcribed recording of an actual remotivation session. The members are ten females from the ages of 68 to 91 who live in a residential-care setting. The session was conducted by a nursing aide trained in a 30-hour remotivation inservice training course. We are presenting a rather lengthy transcription, since we feel that it best represents the back-and-forth movement of the group and the various levels of functioning of each group member. The sensitive awareness of the leader is evident in her handling of the group, and her ability to elicit responses even from the more retiring group members should be noted.

Remotivation Session **Topic—Quilting**

Remotivator: Good morning, Mrs. W. Thank you for coming to the meeting. Good morning, Mrs. A. I'm happy to see you. Mrs. T., welcome. Thank you for coming to the meeting. Miss M., so nice to have you come to our meeting. Mrs. C., I'm glad you could make it. I know it's kind of early to get everybody up. Good morning, Mrs. N.

Mrs. N.: Mary.

Remotivator: May I call you Mary?

Mrs. N.: Oh, yes, everybody calls me Mary.

Remotivator: Okay. I'll do that. Good morning, Mrs. G. Thank you for coming to the meeting.

Mrs. G.: [*Smiles.*]

Miss S.: You don't know my name, I bet!

Remotivator: Oh yes, Miss S., and I'm glad you came this morning. Mrs. F., thank you for coming to the meeting.

Mrs. F.: Thank you for inviting me.

Remotivator: Mrs. E., it's nice to see you. Thank you for coming.

Mrs. E.: I'm glad to be here.

Remotivator: It's kind of warm today, isn't it?

Mrs. G.: It is close, yes.

Remotivator: What kind of activities does a housewife do in the daytime?

Mrs. A.: *Ach du lieber!*

Miss S.: Always housework.

Remotivator: Always housework. Good.

Mrs. T.: Everything.

Remotivator: Everything. Mrs. T. said "everything." Mrs. G., what would a housewife do in the daytime?

Mrs. G.: Cleaning, sweeping.

Remotivator: What did you say, Miss S.?

Miss S.: Housework.

Remotivator: Yes. Housework.

Miss M.: Everything.

Remotivator: That covers a lot of territory!

Miss M.: Yes.

Remotivator: Mary, what would a housewife do in the daytime?

Mrs. N.: Wash, iron, cooking and . . . wait for your husband to come in. [*Laughter.*]

Remotivator: And wait for your husband to come in. That's true. Mrs. G.?

Mrs. G.: Well, she'd start cleaning up the kitchen, the breakfast dishes and all that first.

Remotivator: Yes. That's right.

Mrs. G.: Then she'd start the luncheon and the dinner . . .

Remotivator: And get ready for dinner. And how would she keep busy in the evening?

Miss S.: That's dangerous.
[*Laughter.*]

Remotivator: That's dangerous?

Miss S.: Washing dishes.
[*Laughter.*]

Remotivator: Mrs. F., how would a housewife keep busy in the evening?

Mrs. F.: Sewing, crocheting.

Remotivator: Sewing, crocheting. Yes. Mrs. E.?

Mrs. E.: She cooks supper, turns down the beds . . . listens to the radio.

Mrs. A.: Ya! Ya!

Remotivator: Oh, she's going to have a nice evening. You are not going to put her to work in the evening?
[*Laughter.*]
How would a farm wife spend her evening?

Mrs. A.: Take her shoes and run!

Remotivator: Can anyone else tell me what a farm wife might do in the evening?

Mrs. A.: Begin to despair!

Remotivator: Oh . . . How did women spend their evenings 60 years ago?

Mrs. G.: She might get the babies ready for bed and clean up the kitchen and get ready for the morning.

Remotivator: Yes. All important things.

Miss S.: When my mother finished the work, then she'd go out to her friend's house.

Remotivator: Go visiting. Yes . . . Mrs. F., what would you have done 60 years ago?

Mrs. F.: My mother used to wash and iron and catch up for the next day.

Remotivator: Working and getting ready for the next day. Fine.

Mrs. E.: Sixty years ago, my mother, after she got us up to bed, used to get out the carded wool and spin. Each night she'd get out the spinning wheel and warp it up. She'd work every night on that spinning wheel.

Remotivator: Those were busy evenings. Tell me . . . what kinds of handiwork did women do in a group years ago?

Mrs. E.: In a group?

Mrs. W.: Not in a group. But I did it myself.

Remotivator: You did it yourself? Did anyone else ever do any sewing in a quilting bee?

Mrs. T.: Mm-mm-mm . . . I watched.

Remotivator: I see. Well, you can know a great deal from watching. . . . Miss M. has a poem she'd like to read us on the quilting party.

Miss M: *The Quilting Party*

In the sky the bright stars glittered,
On the bank the pale moon shone,
And it was from Aunt Dinah's quilting party
    I was seeing Nellie home.
On my arm a soft hand rested,
Rested light as ocean foam,
And it was from Aunt Dinah's quilting party
    I was seeing Nellie home.

[*Applause.*]

Remotivator: That was very nice, Miss M. Thank you. Can anyone tell me what a quilt *is*?

Miss S.: A quilt is something that starts with pieces of goods like a patchwork and in between the patches they put cotton.

Remotivator: They put a cotton padding?

Miss S.: A padding.

Remotivator: That's right. . . . How else could we describe a quilt?

Mrs. F.: The only thing I know about it is, it is a pretty bedcover.

Remotivator: Yes. Quilts are bedcovers.

Remotivator: Fine. When do you think quilt-making was invented?

Miss S.: Before my time.

Remotivator: Mrs. C., when do you think quilt-making was invented?

Mrs. C.: Quilt is made of many pieces, putting them together.

Remotivator: Patching them together. That is a type of quilt. When do you think quilt-making was invented . . . Miss M?

Miss M.: I have no idea.

Miss S.: Before my time.

Remotivator: I read that it probably started in Colonial times, when material was hard to get, so women used all the little scraps that they had. . . . Can anyone tell me how quilts are made nowadays?

Mrs. F.: They are made by machinery in the factories.

Remotivator: Yes. They are most often made by machines. That is true. . . . Tell me, what different kinds of quilts are there?

Mrs. N.: There's wool . . .

Mrs. F.: Different kinds of material: wool, cotton; and they put the cotton in between.

Remotivator: Right. Any other type of quilt that you know?

Mrs. A.: A quilt.

Mrs. C.: Small pieces, put together.

Remotivator: What would that be called?

Mrs. C.: A quilt.

Remotivator: There is a special name. Does anyone know what that would be called? Small pieces joined together. What is the name for that type of quilt?

Mrs. E.: A patch quilt.

Remotivator: A patchwork quilt. That's right, Mrs. E. Are they the easiest ones to make?

Mrs. E.: No. I don't think so.

Mrs. W.: No . . . mm-mm-mm . . . Maybe so.

Remotivator: There is more detail in patchwork quilts, Mrs. W?
[*Remotivator picks up small pieces of material.*]
I have a few samples here of the materials that are used in making quilts.

Miss M.: Oh, yes.

Miss S.: Calico.

Remotivator: First you would have just what Miss S. says. What is that, Miss S.?
[*Remotivator holds materials and shows them to each in turn.*]

Miss S.: Calico, isn't it? A cotton . . . ?

Remotivator: A type of cotton. Right.

Mrs. G.: Gingham.

Mrs. F.: A cotton, calico or gingham, more or less.

Remotivator: Gingham and calico are different types of cotton material. These samples are also types of cotton prints. So you would start with just your materials at first?

Mrs. E.: You collect them.

Remotivator: So you collect the pieces. Then what happens after you have your material?

Mrs. T.: Together.

Remotivator: Put them together, Mrs. T.?

Mrs. N.: You can cut them to the size you want.

Remotivator: Right. What else can be made of quilted material, besides bedcovers?
[*Remotivator shows each a set of quilted pot holders made of previously shown materials.*]

Miss S.: Oh yeah! Pot holders, aren't they?

Mrs. F.: They're made like pants!
[*Laughter.*]

Remotivator: Right . . . and they feel heavier. Is there something in between, or is it just cotton material?

Mrs. W.: Let me see.

Mrs. N.: A padding.

Remotivator: Yes. . . . Mrs. C., can you feel the inside?

Mrs. C.: There's padding inside.

Remotivator: You're right. You do feel the padding inside?

Mrs. C.: Yes.

Remotivator: Does all quilting have to have a padding?

Mrs. E.: Yes. Carded wool or cotton. It's all put in on the frame and they have to put in extra. You have to sit down on a stool and sort it out with your hands.

Remotivator: You must have had a lot to do in the evenings.

Mrs. E.: Of course we did.

Remotivator: Can you feel the padding? These are some of the things that were made up in our own therapy department.

Remotivator: [*Shows a quilted mitt with a puppet head.*]

Mrs. W.: A cat?

Remotivator: Yes. It's made to look like a cat.

Mrs. F.: A hot pot mitt!

Remotivator: A hot pot mitt. . . . Miss S., how do you like this? This was also made in our therapy department.

Miss S.: Something to put on your hand when you get a hot pot?

Remotivator: Yes. It would be protection for your hand.

Mrs. G.: I say the same.

Remotivator: Mrs. A., would you like to put it on?

Mrs. A.: Ya! Ya!

Remotivator: You would say the same? That's right. Mary?

Miss M.: For your hand on the hot pots.

Mrs. N.: You could use it for everything . . . baking pot, coffee pot, cooking.

Mrs. F.: And your hands would be always good.

Remotivator: Miss M.?

Miss M.: I wouldn't know what it was.

Remotivator: Would you like to guess?

Miss M.: Some kind of glove.

Remotivator: Some kind of glove. That's right. Mrs. C.?

Mrs. C.: A glove.

Remotivator: Right. To be used for what?

Mrs. C.: To put on.

Remotivator: Mrs. T.?

Mrs. T.: Mm-mm-mm. Not sure.

Remotivator: To wear?

Mrs. G.: That's what it looks like: a mitt.

Mrs. T.: Mm-mm-mm. Yes.

Remotivator: Yes. A mitt. They do these upstairs in the occupational therapy room.

Mrs. E.: Isn't it a skull-cap?

Remotivator: It *looks* like a skull-cap from where you're looking at it. Suppose I put it on my hand?

Mrs. E.: Oh yes.

Remotivator: . . . But it's a mitten.
[*Much simultaneous talking and laughing.*]

Miss M.: Very fancy.

Miss S.: That looks like a puppet!

Remotivator: They made these last year. They sold very well. Yes. It's a mitt, made like a puppet. Did you ever use any of these?
[*More talking, laughing.*]

Mrs. T.: No.

Mrs. W.: I'm not so sure.
[*Laughter.*]
[*Remotivator shows a large section of an unfinished quilt.*]

Mrs. E.: I do. Yes.

Remotivator: That was what you were talking about?

Mrs. E.: Oh yes. It's like a patch and it's quilted . . . cut like a quilt.

Remotivator: That's a quilt. Yes, a portion of it . . . Mrs. F?

Mrs. F.: Pretty quilting.

Remotivator: It's nice and soft.

Miss S.: It has cotton in between.

Remotivator: Yes. It has cotton in between, that's right.

Miss S.: It's pretty. I'd like this for my bureau.

Remotivator: You want to take this for your bureau? I'll have to get permission from Sister. All right?

Miss S.: Okay.

Remotivator: This would be very pretty as a carriage cover. . . . Mrs. C.?

Mrs. C.: Pretty. Yes.

Remotivator: See how soft that is.

Miss M.: It is soft.

Remotivator: Is this what you worked on, Mrs. W.?

Mrs. W.: No. I didn't do this. I made dresses.

Remotivator: I see.

Mrs. W.: But I *could* do that.

Remotivator: You're handy at sewing. I know. . . . Tell me, what color could a quilt be?

Mrs. G.: Any color.

Remotivator: Yes. Any color. What color would make up prettiest, do you think?
[*Many responses: "Blue," "Red," "Pink," "Green," "I like red."*]

Remotivator: Red, blue, pink. You like blue, Mrs. T.?

Mrs. T.: Mm-mm-mm. Yes. Blue is nice.

Remotivator: Miss M.?

Miss M.: Depends on the other colors. I don't know.

Remotivator: What are quilting frames?

Mrs. A.: I don't want to commit myself.

Miss S.: You put the material on them.

Remotivator: All right. Miss S. says that the frames are for the quilt material.

Mrs. E.: They're a long piece of wood, dear, and a narrow piece at the ends, and a certain size, and you have to put both threads in and tie them so they pull stiff as you work through.

Remotivator: To work through. I see . . .

Mrs. E.: You put the material on them.

Mrs. G.: If it had legs, it could stand up, if it had to be put on the floor. I've seen them put on the floor.

Mrs. E.: Yes. They can have legs—a three-legged stool.

Remotivator: And some have legs?

Mrs. E.: Oh, yes. There are two kinds of frames. There was a backing that went into the frame at the same time. Some made the material very stiff, till it was very, very . . . just so.

Remotivator: Yes, I see. How many people could work on a quilt at one time? [*Many responses: "Two," "four," or "five."*]

Mrs. N.: To put it together?

Remotivator: Yes. How many people could work on a quilt at one time, do you think?

Mrs. N.: No more than two.

Remotivator: No more than two. Anyone else?. . . . How many people?

Miss M.: I haven't any idea.

Mrs. C.: About two or three, yeah.

Mrs. G.: It takes a couple to put the frame together.

Mrs. C.: Yeah. Put the frame together.

Remotivator: Just to put the frame together? I see. And what has to be done next?

Mrs. E.: Seat three on both sides, and one on each end. They have different designs. They have a chalk, and they chalk the different designs . . . and the different threads.

Remotivator: Sounds very well planned.

Mrs. E.: And it comes out pretty.

Remotivator: What kinds of needles are used?

Mrs. G.: Darning ones.

Mrs. E.: Quilting needles. They'd be best. Yes.

Mrs. F.: A large needle.

Remotivator: Are bone needles used or a steel needle?

Mrs. G.: No. It's a steel needle.

Remotivator: And what special stitches are used?

Mrs. E.: Any special.

Mrs. G.: Sometimes a buttonhole stitch, sometimes a hemming stitch.

Remotivator: Buttonhole or hemming stitches. Do you think . . . ?

Mrs. E.: A chain stitch or a cable stitch.

Remotivator: Many different kinds. . . . Mrs. F., what did you say?

Mrs. F.: A running stitch.

Remotivator: I see. . . . Was that all done by hand or by machine?

Mrs. E.: By hand.

Mrs. F.: By hand.

Remotivator: How many pieces, or swatches, of material have to be cut?

Miss S.: According to the frame.

Mrs. C.: According to the size. . . .

Mrs. N.: Well, depends on the size.

Miss S.: All different sizes.

Remotivator: Measuring it first is important. . . . How long do you think it would take to make the quilt?

Mrs. G.: Months.

Miss S.: According to how many times you work on it.

Remotivator: Certainly. The number of times you work on it . . .

Mrs. G.: According to how many people are working on it.

Remotivator: That's true. Mary, what do you think?

Mrs. N.: If you have a small one, it takes less time to put it together. A small quilt or a big one . . .

Remotivator: Yes. It depends on the size. . . . Who has ever seen one made or helped to make one?

Mrs. G.: I have.

Mrs. E.: I did.

Remotivator: You've both had lots of experience.

Mrs. E.: Always a patch quilt.

Mrs. G.: I made it by patches, too.

Remotivator: Patchwork quilts, mostly? Is there anyone else that helped to make one? Miss M. . . . No? . . . You never did, Mrs. C.? You must have, in Venezuela!

Mrs. C.: They make it, but I didn't . . . I watch it. Little pieces and so . . .

Remotivator: So you have seen them made . . . In what areas of the country do you think quilting is still done?

Mrs. G.: In the West. That's where we sent ours after we got them done, to have them quilted.

Mrs. G.: They do wonderful work on them.

Remotivator: In what area of the country do you think quilting is still done?

Mrs. F.: I think in the West.

Remotivator: In the West?

Miss S.: I think any place.

Remotivator: I think that's true, perhaps in some farming areas of the country.

Mrs. E.: They do it in Ireland yet.

Remotivator: Oh, they still do it in Ireland?

Mrs. E.: They make the long thread, and . . .
[*Takes a long pause.*]
. . . save the material for it, and then they have both sides quilted so you can turn it any way.

Remotivator: Reversible?

Mrs. E.: Yes.

Remotivator: Tell me . . . if you ladies were invited to a quilting bee, what job would you prefer?

Mrs. C.: I watch!

Remotivator: Oh!

Miss S.: I'd take the frame.

Remotivator: You'd take the frame? Fine. What job would you like, Mrs. F., if you were invited to a quilting bee?

Mrs. F.: Sew the patches together.

Remotivator: Good. You'd sew the patches together . . . Mrs. E., if you were invited to a quilting bee, what job would you like?

Mrs. E.: Patches are not so good, 'cause they're all going to do something of that, no matter what part they'd be working on, and I'd be nervous about how it was all getting together, so it wouldn't be useless.

Remotivator: Putting it together . . . you would like fitting it into the chalked design?

Mrs. E.: Yes. It is very interesting.

Remotivator: Mrs. W., if you were invited to a quilting bee, what part of the work would you like to do?

Mrs. W.: I don't know.

Remotivator: You wouldn't know?

Mrs. W.: I don't know anything about the making of a quilt.

Remotivator: But you said you'd like to do sewing.

Mrs. W.: If that job is vacant, but there's lots of others, like myself, you know. [*Laughs.*]

Remotivator: Well, if you were the first one there, maybe you'd get the plain sewing part of it.

Mrs. E.: I think the hemming is very interesting too.

Remotivator: The hemming?

Mrs. E.: The hemming and knotting them together. Many times you'd change to different things at the party.

Remotivator: And do a little of each part of the work.

Mrs. E.: Yes.

Remotivator: Mrs. A., would you like to work on sewing a quilt?

Mrs. A.: No. No . . .

Remotivator: That doesn't interest you? There are other things you might like to do?

Mrs. A.: [*Laughs.*]

Remotivator: Mrs. T., what part would you like, if you were invited?

Mrs. T.: Mm-mm-mm. Maybe crochet.

Remotivator: You would just want to crochet one?

Mrs. T.: Mm-mm-mm. Maybe.

Remotivator: That's good, I'll take the one you crochet!
[*Laughs.*]
Miss M.?

Miss M.: Make the design.

Remotivator: You like to arrange the designs for the quilt, that's nice. . . . And Mary?

Mrs. N.: I'm making one now, so gotta make first the patches, and then put them together.

Remotivator: Yes. What part would you like to do if you were invited? What would you like to do best?

Miss N.: The patches.

Remotivator: Well, That's good. I hope we get a nice quilt out of that!
[*Laughter.*]

Mrs. E.: When I first came to this country, I brought some warm quilting.

Remotivator: You brought some from the old country?

Mrs. E.: Coming out here in 1906, I brought them from my aunt.

Remotivator: That's nice. Do you still have any of those that you worked on?

Mrs. E.: Ah, no, I haven't. Right now, I haven't any.

Remotivator: Your daughter doesn't have any?

Mrs. E.: I have a patch quilt I made since. I have a very nice one. Specially cut and shaped.

Remotivator: Oh, I'm sorry, I didn't know. If I had known, I would have asked you, or had your daughter bring it in, so we could have shown it.

Mrs. E.: Sure, that's all right.

Remotivator: Well, I have really heard a great many things about quilts I never knew. So much work and thought has to go into handmade quilts. I guess that's why they are so beautiful and so prized. I enjoyed talking about quilts with all of you today. Okay, Mrs. E., thank you for coming to the meeting today. You were very interesting.

Mrs. E.: T'was very nice.

Remotivator: Mrs. W., next time we'll talk about dresses. I think you will enjoy that more.

Mrs. W.: [*Laughs.*]
That's for another time.

Remotivator: Mrs. A., thank you for coming this morning. I hope you enjoyed it.

Mrs. A.: [*Laughs.*]

Remotivator: Mrs. T., thank you for coming to the meeting.

Mrs. T.: [*Smiles and shakes head.*]

Remotivator: We should have had your daughter bring in the quilt you crocheted.

Mrs. T.: Mmm-mm-mm.

Remotivator: Maybe she can bring it in another time.

Mrs. T.: No. She's away.

Remotivator: She's on vacation? When she comes back. Mrs. C., thank you for coming to the meeting.

Mrs. C.: Yeah. I like.

Remotivator: Miss M., thank you for coming and for reading the poem. It was very nice. We all enjoyed it.

Remotivator: Mary, thank you so much for coming. I'll be looking forward to seeing your quilt when it's finished.

Mrs. N.: My pleasure.

Remotivator: Mrs. G., thank you for coming, and for all the information you gave.

Mrs. G.: Okay.

Remotivator: Thank you. . . .

Miss S.: Maybe we'll make a quilt now!
[*Laughs.*]

Remotivator: Okay, we'll do that. Mrs. G., want to make a quilt?

Mrs. G.: Yes.

Remotivator: Fine.

Miss S.: When you have the time. . . .

Remotivator: Mrs. F., thank you. It was a pleasure to have you here. . . . We'll plan to meet next Wednesday at ten o'clock, since I'm off next Tuesday. Okay? . . . and maybe we'll talk about dresses and fashions. How about that?
[*Affirmative response from several.*]
In the meantime, I can speak to Sister in O.T. upstairs, and she can help those who want to work on quilts. Okay? See you next Wednesday.

QUESTIONS AND ANSWERS ABOUT REMOTIVATION THERAPY

Is Remotivation a Form of Psychotherapy? No. Remotivation usually deals with noncontroversial topics—topics that are objective instead of subjective. Discussions center around realities of everyday life and use topics such as holidays, nature, fashion, current events, birds, hats, food, and history. The technique focuses on the "unwounded" areas of the personality, leaving the "wounded" areas for psychotherapists to deal with.

Even If We Deal with Objective Topics, Don't Some of These Involve Sensitive Areas and Feelings? Yes, but the remotivator, generally not a trained psychotherapist, accepts what is said by the patient without exploring the feelings involved. For example, at one session, when Christmas was being discussed, one woman began to cry. She told the group that her husband had died on Christmas Day. The remotivator expressed her sorrow over the woman's loss and then continued the session, which was on Christmas foods. The woman stopped crying and joined in the discussion, focusing on the special foods that she had cooked that her husband had enjoyed. A trained psychotherapist may be asked to see this patient later in order to explore the feelings that she expressed during the remotivation session.

What Topics Are Not Used in Remotivation Sessions? In general, such topics as death, religion, love, sex, and politics are not used. However, it has been found that, in some facilities, aged individuals have had stimulating discussions on controversial topics, such as the generation gap, politics, and remarriage. The remotivator should use his or her sensitivity in deciding if a particular group would benefit from discussions dealing with more controversial topics.

If Remotivation Is Just a Discussion Group, Why Does It Require a Special Technique? Because it is designed to meet the special needs of those who need more stimulation to promote interaction with others. The technique thus places the remotivator physically in the center of the group, where he or she can move about freely to lead or dominate the action by providing extra stimulation. There is a definite framework used in order to develop the discussion topic. The technique also focuses on just one topic instead of several; the discussion group does not meet merely to socialize. In summary, remotivation therapy is a structured, primarily leader-dominated discussion technique that explores an objective topic.

Are Compliments Important? Can't the Group Members Interpret Them As Being False and Insincere? Compliments are a form of reinforcement through which specific behaviors are encouraged. Instead of being insincere, the remotivator uses positive comments with which he or she is comfortable. For example, remotivators have found that calling attention to the way that a particular resident's hair may look after a trip to the beauty parlor or commenting on an attractive dress that someone is wearing are statements that are often received with pleasure. Each remotivator should take special care to include each person so that no one will feel neglected. Compliments may also include some factual information that the individual would like to share, such as the fact that "Mrs. N. has just become a great-grandparent." The remotivator who knows the residents uses such available knowledge in the meeting as a way of enhancing this total climate of acceptance.

If We Include a Couple of Confused Residents in the Group, Don't We Run Into Objections By the Other Group Members? That may happen. If the behavior of the more confused person leads to rejection by the others, plans should be made to redesign the group and to place the confused person elsewhere. If the person's behavior is disruptive, and if the remotivator's attempts to focus the patient's attention are not effective, the remotivator may have to remove the person from the group for the remainder of that session. Group members will often act in a protective way, however, trying to explain to the confused person what is being said, giving the person the "right answer." If this happens, one of the direct goals of remotivation is being met—that of stimulating interaction.

During one session, the authors watched a confused resident stand up and move her chair back, as though to walk away. The remotivator stopped and said, "I hope you can stay with us, Mrs. B." But the resident said "no" and wandered out of the room. The discussion continued and, a short time later, the woman returned and sat down again. The remotivator commented, "I'm so glad to have you back, Mrs. B. You were missed." The remotivator then continued as though nothing had happened. Residents should not be forced to attend remotivation sessions. Instead, they should be encouraged and invited to come back again.

Do Remotivation Sessions Always Start with Questions? Sometimes the remotivator can use a poem that leads into the topic. This is actually the way remotivation began, by reading poetry and asking questions. For example, "Trees" by Joyce Kilmer could lead into the topic of beauty. Sometimes a newspaper item or a quotation can be used, but this depends on the level of the group.

Does It Matter What Kind of Poetry Is Used? Yes. The poem should be simple, objective, and appropriate to the topic. It should be rhythmic and it should rhyme. If it is well-read, poetry is generally received with pleasure. Residents often applaud at the end to indicate their pleasure. Gloomy, depressing poems or those difficult to understand should not be used.

What Do You Do When You Cannot Find a Poem That Fits the Topic? One way would be to start with a related poem that could lead into the topic. Another way would be to use a poem that merely mentions the topic. Still another way would be to write your own poetry.

Are There Other Ways of Giving Rewards Besides Using Compliments? Yes. Other forms include using one's smile, having a warm facial expression, and using eye contact. Verbal reinforcements such as "yes," "that's true," and "fine" are also rewards and encourage further contributions from group members.

What Do You Do If Someone In the Group Gives An Incorrect Answer? Honest feedback should be given for incorrect information. If the remotivator feels that the group member did not hear the question, he or she may simply rephrase or repeat the question. If the response is still incorrect, the correct answer is provided by saying, for example, "Easter is a spring holiday," or by asking another group member, trying in that way to elicit a correct answer.

Does the Remotivator Need to Know a Lot About the Topic Being Used? He or she does not need to be an expert but is expected to review basic information before the session starts.

Where Can One Find the Information Needed For a Remotivation Session? Good sources of information are newspaper articles; magazine clippings; stories and pictures about such famous people as inventors, soldiers, painters, and movie stars; and articles on soap making, stamp collecting, printing, television shows, movies, and many others. Coworkers and other remotivators are good resources. Library materials, such as encyclopedias and dictionaries, may also be consulted.

Where Does the Remotivator Get All Of the Necessary Props? Props for the session may be obtained from departments in the remotivator's own facility, including the recreation-therapy, occupational-therapy, and dietary departments. Items that leaders or other people have collected may also be used.

Do Residents Ask Questions During the Meeting? Yes. Usually, the remotivator throws the question out to the group first. It has been found that someone usually comes up with an answer but, if no one does, the remotivator supplies the answer. If a group member asks a question that no one, including the remotivator, can answer, the remotivator may say, "Mrs. S. had a very good question. Since none of us knows the answer, perhaps we can look it up later and let everyone know." The promise, once made, is always kept, and the information, once collected, is shared with the group.

Does the Remotivator Ever Have a Session In Which the Group Does Not Respond? That seldom happens. When individuals do not respond spontaneously, however, the remotivator should direct a specific question to one of the residents; for example, "Mrs. S., what other things could people do to celebrate July 4th besides watch a parade?" Many times, a withdrawn resident participates just by remaining in a group and by observing and listening to what is happening. This is accepted, but the resident should be encouraged to participate more fully.

Do Residents Ever Get Into Arguments In the Session? Yes, some residents interact by being argumentative. When the remotivator sees difficulties occurring that tend to foster disruption in the group, she or he can intervene just as when the group strays from the topic or when an overly talkative resident monopolizes a session. For example, the remotivator can introduce a summarizing comment and then redirect the group's attention to the next idea.

Do Residents Enjoy the Sessions? Remotivators have stated that residents genuinely enjoy the sessions. It has been observed that they talk about a session for days after it has taken place with other residents, staff, family members, and visitors.

Can the Remotivator Offer His or Her Own Comments In a Session? It is very important for the remotivator to feel a part of the group, and it has been found that the remotivator who adds comments of her or his own often enhances the interaction of the group. However, this does not mean using the leadership role to monopolize the conversation; the remotivator should interact but should not take over.

How Do Remotivators Feel About the Technique? In general, remotivators have expressed deep feelings of satisfaction and personal reward from their experiences leading remotivation sessions. They have reported that the information they learned from the residents during a session helped them to understand these residents as individuals who have varied backgrounds and experiences. Remotivators have also reported that they were not aware that they could be group leaders and were delighted to find that they could be effective group leaders to whom others responded. They stated that the technique enhanced their own feelings of self-esteem and self-satisfaction.

CHARTING PROGRESS

In order to keep an accurate record of a patient's progress, patient behavior should be charted after each remotivation session (see Appendix D). The remotivator observes the effects of the session on each patient's behavior—the interaction of the patients while in the group setting—then records this information when the session has ended. Accurate records maintained over several months will indicate how well each patient is progressing in the group.

On the evaluation form, we have suggested that the remotivator check the number corresponding most closely to a patient's response to the task described during *that particular session only*. If the patient has usually participated in the day's session, the remotivator would check "2" as the appropriate rating. If, however, the patient seemed to participate only "sometimes" during that session, his or her rating would be "1." The patient's level of enjoyment is rated in the same way. The form is filled out in *triplicate*; one copy is for the medical chart (placed there at the end of a month), one is for the remotivator, and one is for the remotivator's supervisor.

In order to determine the general effect of the remotivation program, the remotivator might ask other staff members if they have noticed any different kinds of behavior in a patient since she or he started remotivation or since the last few sessions. The remotivator then could use this information in subsequent sessions. For example, if a patient had not been generally helpful to others and now appears to be helpful, the remotivator might enlist this patient's aid in helping other patients, such as helping to move wheelchair patients. A consistent scoring of "2" ("usually") would indicate that the patient could be ready for a higher-level group, such as an open-ended, nonstructured discussion group; group therapy; art therapy; and others.

REFERENCE NOTES

1. Busse, E. W., & Blazer, D. G., (Eds.). *Handbook of geriatric psychiatry*. New York: Van Nostrand Reinhold Co., 1980, p. 458.
2. Barnes, E. K., Sack, A., & Shore, H. Guidelines to treatment approaches. *The Gerontologist*, 1973, *13*, 513–527.
3. Ibid., p. 518.
4. Isaacs, A. D., & Post, F. (Eds.). *Studies in geriatric psychiatry*. New York: Wiley, 1978, p. 258.
5. American Psychiatric Association. *Remotivation technique: A manual for use in nursing homes*. Washington, D.C., no date.

9

Implementation of the Stepladder Approach

OVERALL GOALS

No matter what the modality, the primary goal of the techniques that we have discussed is to keep all patients functioning at their optimal level. Since all patients are individuals and, therefore, are always functioning at a variety of levels, there is a possibility for a wide range of goals. The patient who is acutely ill with a stroke may seem to respond as confusion lifts and may eventually be rehabilitated to his or her own home, but the frail elderly person who has long-standing chronic brain syndrome may show confusion that will never decrease. For the former, there will be promotion from one modality to another—from sensory training to reality orientation to remotivation and perhaps eventual return to the community. The latter patient will most likely be maintained for an extended period of time in a sensory or reality group.

Basic to all modalities is the goal of increasing interpersonal skills and the number and quality of interactions. For the most regressed patients, this may mean 'only' the re-establishment of eye contact after many seemingly nonproductive sessions. For others, there may be a rapid improvement in grooming habits as a result of group participation. For some, there may be an incentive for independence in the activities of daily living (ADL); if residents want to get to group meetings, they will be more attentive to dressing themselves. Certain residents will become more cognizant of others' needs; in time, one resident may choose to wheel a wheelchair-bound roommate to the sessions. All of the above may be instrumental in maintaining or possibly raising self-esteem and in minimizing apathy, withdrawal, and even depression.

It must be remembered that, for the residents involved, rehabilitation potentials and goals are often limited. We must also remember, however, that even small successes can improve the quality of life in the closed environment of the institution. Remember also that programs may appear childlike but still be rehabilitative.

SETTING UP THE STEPLADDER APPROACH

The leader who is to conduct each of the stepladder therapies should be one who is familiar with the patients on the unit. In many cases, since other staff members will be involved in the implementation of these techniques, some of them should be involved when possible. In setting up, as in following through, we encourage and stress the team approach. When the senior author was consultant to nursing home staff, this was used with optimal results. The leader for the designated technique chose patients in conjunction with the nurse clinician. Together, they selected patients suitable for each level, asking questions of themselves and of each other that would be specific to each of the techniques. For example, as we mentioned earlier, in choosing patients for sensory training, both would look for patients who would respond to sensory stimulation but who were not sufficiently aware to respond to reality orientation. A simple: "Do you think Mrs. B. would be right for sensory training?", when asked of two knowledgeable staff members, is more likely to elicit an accurate answer than if one alone were to make the judgment. Similarly, patients for reality orientation and remotivation were so selected. What also needs to be considered is the patient's schedule for other hospital-related activities in order to ensure that activities and sessions do not overlap. In addition, if staff is aware that the time designated for sensory training is a time when the patient receives daily or once-weekly steady visits from family members, this should also be taken into account and some other time chosen.

GROUP ATTENDANCE

Once the groups have been set up, they are held in as consistent a manner as possible. This should be true whether all members are present or only a few. When there are only a few, it is good to begin the session by mentioning this fact, such as: "I see that Mrs. J. and Mrs. L. are not with us today. I understand that Mrs. J. is not feeling well and that Mrs. L. has a visitor. We will miss them but will continue with our group and hope that they join us the next time."

This type of verbalization is made at the beginning of each stepladder modality, even if it seems likely that members are little aware of their missing peers. This same is true if a peer has died. Mention is made of this fact, with appropriate empathic comments, before the formal session begins, allowing for members' responses, if they are forthcoming. Again, this is done whether or not it is the group leader's understanding that "nobody noticed."

The ability to verbalize a feeling, such as "I am sad that Mrs. P. has died," and the fact that the person will be missed, on some level, are not the same. Emotions, or just a sensing that "something is amiss," may take place within the patient without the ability to communicate this. It is the group leader's responsibility to relate these facts of reality to the group in an empathic way. While leaders need to have the qualities of sensitivity, empathy, ability to communicate with patients, motivation, and the like, as general qualities, there are (nonetheless) differences among people that need to be respected.

MATCHING THE GROUP LEADER TO THE TECHNIQUE

Not only do patients vary, in that each should be assigned a particular therapeutic modality based upon the team's estimation of his or her need, but each group leader or therapeutic agent also varies in personal style and preference. Since sensory training is a technique that requires a great deal of touch contact with the patient, it is helpful to recruit staff who can touch patients with ease. If a group leader cannot touch patients without feeling uncomfortable, he or she should be encouraged to lead one of the other techniques, such as reality-orientation or remotivation therapy. Reality orientation (as discussed in Chapter 7) emphasizes an approach that is mostly verbal. The remotivation technique (discussed in Chapter 8) is most akin to a formal classroom structure. It has been found that leaders who have difficulty with sensory training because they are not comfortable with touch do very well in a technique such as remotivation, which does not require close physical contact with patients. Every technique requires that the leader and the group establish rapport and that the leader like what she or he is doing and is empathic toward the group members. Group leaders should, therefore, whenever possible, choose the technique with which they are most comfortable; both patients and leaders benefit most from this endeavor. A way of determining which technique seems most "natural" is for each leader to try them all and to choose the one that most suits her or his own style of relating to others.

THE TEAM APPROACH

Most basic to all of the techniques is *consistence*. This can be maintained only if everyone who interacts with the resident is aware of what is going on with this person in terms of level of functioning and assigned treatment approach. Again, this is most easily accomplished by using a team approach. *Everyone* who interacts with the resident, on any level, must be alerted to the fact that the patient is, for example, in a sensory-training group and must be related to with that information in mind. This includes, not only professional and paraprofessional ward personnel, but others (such as housekeeping and maintenance staff).

Team meetings should be held regularly and should include all staff who interact with the resident in order to inform them periodically of the patient's progress. There should be a team leader who knows the residents well and who is able to maintain the team's cohesiveness. The leader should keep everyone informed of the patient's progress and should have all team members discuss problems and seek solutions. Such a leader may be a nurse, social worker, activities worker, or perhaps an aide or an orderly.

Remember that the various treatment programs outlined in this book are not to be perceived as limited programs occurring on a particular day for a limited period of time. Instead, they are to be considered as *approaches* to the resident. In other words, if a patient is in a sensory-training or reality-orientation group for a limited amount of time several times a week, the *approach* of sensory training should be an ongoing, 24-hour-a-day approach. This patient should be touched as often as possible and afforded as many opportunities as possible in order to develop his or her ability to discriminate stimuli. This approach should be used, not only during group sessions, but also throughout the entire day by everyone who comes in contact with the patient. To be most consistent, staff from the recreation-therapy and occupational-therapy departments should also be made aware that this sensory-training patient needs to have special attention paid to her or his inability to differentiate different textures, smells, or tastes.

FAMILY INVOLVEMENT

Members of the patient's family should be informed about the technique to which their aging family member has been assigned, and the technique should be thoroughly explained to them. They should be told that the technique is a total approach to be used by all persons who interact with the patient in any way. They should be asked to relate to the patient in a similar fashion and should be considered as adjunct staff. If their family member is in a sensory-training group, for example, the rationale for this should be explained to them, the technique should be described, and they should be asked to use this approach in their interactions with the patient. They should be encouraged to touch the patient whenever possible and to offer the patient various opportunities to develop discriminatory capacities for different kinds of sensory experiences. For example, when a family member visits, he or she could offer the patient an orange and ask how it tastes, if the patient likes it, or what it tastes like—is it sweet, very juicy, a little too tangy? This could easily be included in normal conversation and would prove very helpful to the total approach. It has also been found that, when family members are involved, their morale increases, because they feel that something is being done for their aging family member and, most important, that they themselves are part of the therapeutic process. In addition, they are less prone to feeling that these techniques are too childlike. Family members should also be informed of the patient's progress so that they are aware of how he or she is really functioning at different points.

The authors know of one family member, a wife, who was kept informed of her husband's progress in remotivation therapy. She also visited at various times while he was in session and was allowed to sit at some distance and observe him and the group (with the patient's approval). After some time, she decided to take her husband home to live. She explained that, if she had not observed him during remotivation sessions and seen behaviors that she had no longer thought possible, she would never have concluded that he could function at home. Involving the wife in her husband's rehabilitation may have done much to restimulate her interest in taking him home again and may have uplifted her morale to the point where she felt that she could care for him again in their home surroundings.

RELATIONSHIP OF STIMULATION TECHNIQUES TO PSYCHOTHERAPY

Therapy may be considered that which is beneficial to others. Stimulation techniques may be considered a form of therapy, but they are not the same as psychotherapy. Traditional psychotherapy is a form of treatment that is intrapsychic in nature. The client's behaviors and current functioning level are explored in terms of past experiences and how they relate to the way that the patient functions at the present time; that is, what gets in the way of the patient's ability to function better. The therapist tries to give the client some insight into his or her inner life and helps the patient to learn not to "trip over his own feet."

Stimulation techniques, although therapeutic in the broad sense, are not psychotherapy because the therapist, or group leader, does not explore the dynamics of the personality or make any interpretations. Instead, he or she stays with the limited goals of each technique being used. In addition, where *cure* is often the goal of the person who seeks traditional psychotherapy, this is not the goal of stimulation techniques. The goal is for the patient to be able to function on a higher level whenever possible; that is, to go from a sensory-training group to a reality-orientation group, or (if this is not possible) to stay in the original group but perhaps not regress further. The thinking here is that the stimulation of the group experience may retard or hold constant any natural regression that might take place more easily if there were no group exposure.

Some forms of psychotherapy (e.g., analytic) place much emphasis on *transference*, the way in which the patient relates to the therapist as he or she once did to other significant figures earlier in life, but this is not the focus of the stimulation techniques. There is no doubt, nevertheless, that every group member does relate to the group leader in a special way—the way in which she or he has related to others in leadership positions. But the group leader of these techniques does not verbalize any such awareness while interacting with the group. The leader should make a mental note of the special way that each group member relates to him or her and should use this (and all information gathered about each patient) for the patient's benefit.

If a patient is particularly hostile toward the group leader, it is possible that some of the patient's early life experiences with people in positions of authority were so negative that the patient reacts with hostility to others in positions of leadership today. The group leader should discuss such observations with the stepladder-approach team. The team may then wish to suggest activities to increase such patients' sense of self-esteem—assign them to some leader-type roles or involve them in discussion groups. The group leader should be aware of patients' responses to the leader and of his or her responses to each patient. This information should then be shared with other team members.

A sensitive awareness of each patient by the group leader is presented in the following description:

> [*A group had just started when one disoriented woman rose to leave the room.*]

Mrs. K.: I have to go home now to feed my kids.

Group leader: Mrs. K., you can't go home. Your children are not there. You now live in a home for older people—the XYZ Nursing Home.

Mrs. K.: I know that. Don't be stupid. That's why I have to leave. Right now. I have to go to my *own home to feed my kids*.

The group leader writes: "No amount of presentation of reality could convince Mrs. K. She felt useless in *the home*. She wanted her own home. She wanted her own role as mother of three children. She wanted to feel useful. She wanted to be wanted by someone she loved!"[1] While the group leader may not have expressed these thoughts directly to the patient, as one might do in traditional psychotherapy, her sensitive awareness, shared with other staff, can be used to help the patient in a therapeutic way.

LIFESTYLE AND THE INSTITUTION

In describing the preceding techniques, we have focused on a group of institutionalized aged who have common characteristics, symptoms, and maladaptations, particularly in the interpersonal sphere. The most common characteristic was regression, although the degree of regression varies. Similarly, there was variation in the amount of social interaction. Patients were therefore categorized and matched to a technique best-suited to their level of functioning.

There are, however, other forms of activity that may also be therapeutic for the aged residing within an institution. In order to be able to best match the activity to the patient, a thorough understanding of the patient's life-long style of functioning is critical.

Although there is a tendency to group all adults over the age of 65 together, as though they were perfectly homogeneous in all aspects, age is only one variable that defines them. Each is a unique individual, continuing in their older years the lifestyles that were theirs when they were younger. The term *lifestyle* itself, coined by Alfred Adler, is defined as "one's characteristic pattern of movement. . . . It includes a unique method of perceiving, conceptualizing, behaving, and striving toward a subjectively determining goal."[2] Each individual, then, is different from all others.

Since there is a continuity of personality structure, the professional who works with the aging adult cannot view each patient in terms of his or her current situation only; instead, this person's way of interacting with the environment is a reflection of past ways of coping—behaviors learned throughout her or his life. The whole person is also more than the sum of all parts and cannot be explained by focusing on a part of that person, such as a current disability. Although the disability does influence the person's social, emotional, and physical ways of coping, the total person determines the meaning that this current ailment has to him or her.

Personnel who work with the aging person must have some awareness of his or her particular lifestyle. This gives them clues to the person's pattern of movement, such as the ways in which he or she perceives, thinks, feels, and acts toward the environment. Included are particular biases, unique points of view, and special "colored glasses" used for perceiving and interpreting events.

To illustrate this concept of picking up cues from the patient, let us look at a situation that was observed in a nursing home. Many patients were sitting around, involved in what may be termed the *doing nothing* syndrome—staring off into space while sitting in their wheelchairs or vacuously watching the blaring television as they sat somewhat near each other (but in no way involved) on benches along the side of the large dayroom or in front of the TV. Suddenly, an aging female patient, dressed similarly to the others (housedress with slippers), came into the room. As she deftly manipulated her walker along the floor, she called out orders to the other patients in a strident, dominant voice, "You there—move over there. You, I told you to sit in that other chair before, so get into it. You now—push your wheelchair closer to her," and so on. A staff member soon came in and brusquely ordered her out of the dayroom. Cursing and mumbling to herself, the patient was eased out by the staff member.

Although this patient's behavior was aggressive, it suggested that this person had some sense of order and a need to control by "doing something" that would permit her to exercise this control. Instead of whisking her out of the room, the staff member should have recognized the need underlying the overt behavior and should have catered to it by moving the behavior in a positive direction. This patient could have been used to sort laundry or organize the seating arrangements of an anticipated bingo game, movie night, or birthday party. In other words, her need to organize, manipulate, and control others should have been diverted toward a positive way of behaving that would have benefited other patients, staff, and (most important) herself. When this was not done, it should have been anticipated that this patient's behavior would continue, to no one's benefit and to everyone's detriment.

REFERENCE NOTES

1. Feil, N. Group work with disoriented nursing home residents. In S. Saul (Ed.), *Group work with the frail elderly*. New York: The Haworth Press, 1983, 59.
2. Croake, J. W. An Adlerian view of life style. *Journal of Clinical Psychology*, 1975, *31*, 513–518.

10

Additional Therapeutic Approaches

ACTIVITIES/RECREATION THERAPY

Another way of dealing with individual behaviors in the institutional setting and helping clients to function at maximum potential is through activities therapy.[1] Paul Haun, one of the authorities writing on recreation, states that recreation is a "primary need of all people."[2] Other authors have consistently stated that recreational activity adds greatly to the general "physical and mental vigor of the resident."[3] Most often, the aging person is not involved in seeking out a recreational activity that she or he would like to pursue. More often than not, activities are imposed by the administration, and choices are either minimal or nonexistent. This stripping away of choice mitigates the fostering of continuity with one's former lifestyle. Avedon suggests that

> . . . recreation is generated from within oneself—another person may act as a catalyst, a specific object or act may have an attracting valence quality, but no force outside the self can make a person experience recreation.[4]

Recreation should be one of the areas within the institution where the patient has a choice, choosing both whether to participate in any activities at all and *which* activities to attend. In the institution, as in the community, recreation serves as a way of improving the quality of life.

Using this as a theoretical underpinning for recreational service, the worker must understand the different types of personality so that the worker can fit the client's personality and the activity. The person who is now a resident of an institution but who never played cards and has no desire to do so should not be pressured into playing cards. The resident who was not socially gregarious in earlier years is not likely to become so now, particularly in the institutional setting.

"Rehabilitative" settings that are truly rehabilitative work toward this goal of allowing and fostering independence in the resident. Recreation, a means of achieving this goal, must be designed to offer the widest range and variety of opportunities. Residents must be encouraged, not only to make choices but also to make decisions that would affect them. Recreation should be a way of both strengthening residents' contact with reality and encouraging the use of their particular abilities and skills. In this way, residents are involved in creating their own human environment.

Planning an Activities Program

In planning any program of activities, it is necessary to remember the essential ingredient: the individual personality of the aging person. One's choice of leisure activities is an aspect of one's personality. In studies, it has been found that there was remarkably little change in *choice* of leisure activities as related to age (ages chosen ranged from 40 to 70 years). It was found that the significance of the leisure activity was more closely related to personality than to age, sex, or social class.[5] The amount and style of an aged person's participation are extensions of patterns begun in childhood and shaped in adulthood. Persons who are active throughout the lifespan will retain this style in their later years, although activity levels may be modified by alterations in life situations, such as physical limitations. For example, the older person may become slower and less agile and thus may be unable to continue to play 18 holes of golf; 9 holes may suffice, or just teeing off on a lawn may be realistic. When even this is impossible, he or she may have to be content to watch golf matches on television. The point is that people generally do not become active or sedentary in later life; instead, they *continue* doing what they have done *all of their lives*.[6]

Recreation Activities

Below is a list of the recreation activities that are often included in activities programs at various residential facilities. This is in no way a complete list but is intended as a guide. The important factor to remember is that there should be activities offered from all of the following categories:

1. *Individual activities*
   - Crossword puzzles (large print, if available)
   - Jigsaw puzzles
   - Reading
   - Television viewing
   - Creative writing
   - Visiting with relatives, friends, or volunteers
   - Photography
   - Knitting
   - Crocheting
   - Sewing
   - Painting
   - Crafts

2. *Small-group activities*

Current-events discussion	Reality orientation
Documentary movies	Remotivation
Dramatics	Group therapy
Body-movement workshop	Residents' council
Music-appreciation group	Crafts
Men's and women's clubs	Choral group
Bible discussion	"Around-the-world" club
Poetry group	Trips
Political-action group	Cards and games
Gourmet club	Dance and art therapy
Sensory training	

3. *Large-group activities*

Feature films	Trips
Garden parties	Birthday parties
Wine-and-cheese parties	Bingo
Picnics	Holiday celebrations
Cocktail parties	Entertainment

4. *Religious activities*

Services—regularly scheduled, e.g., Protestant, Catholic, Jewish	Clergy visits Holiday observances Ethnic celebrations

Individual Activities. Individual activities are engaged in by all residents, whether formally or informally. Many residents may obtain reading and handiwork material from family and friends, but for others, obtaining these items may serve as the first step in establishing rapport between the resident and the activities staff. The possibilities for activities are, of course, unlimited, and the worker must be guided by the residents' skills and interests. Volunteers can be most effective in introducing and guiding individual activities.

When the institutionalized resident is sitting alone, he or she is often pushed to join an activity. It has been suggested, however, that there is a need for some aged people to have opportunities to develop the art of aloneness. Being alone can be enjoyable if it is a *voluntary* aloneness. The person who works with the aged must decide (again, by observing behavior and by talking with the patient) whether the need to be alone is a lifestyle to be respected or whether the patient feels lonely and wishes to become involved. If the latter is the case, the worker should be there to help with that task.[7]

Small-Group Activities. Small-group activities should be developed when there are several residents who have similar interests—a dramatics club, a choral group, a poetry-reading group, or regularly scheduled offerings that may not necessarily attract the same residents each time, including documentary films, current events, discussions, and trips. Small-group activities are the core of a well-planned activities program because they necessitate the active involvement of the resident. Involvement and interest mitigate apathy, withdrawal, and possibly depression.

The number and type of these activities will vary from time to time, according to the interests, education, and skills of the resident population and the availability of appropriate activity leaders. Special-interest groups may be led by interested and capable residents or volunteers, as well as by activities leaders or other staff. For example, in a facility in which the activities staff is all female, the men's club could be led by a male administrator or other male staff member. A language class could be conducted by a bilingual resident. An interested nurse may wish to lead a "Keep-Well Club," or the chef may guide the "Gourmet Club." Small groups may also be created to accommodate the interest of community groups. If the local garden club wishes to present a few sessions on flower arranging, this can be easily integrated into the schedule.

A few words of caution: There may be some residents who may participate only in small groups or only in a few individual activities. They may be reluctant to mingle in crowds because they may feel that they do not "fit in" with everyone or because they may have very specific interests and needs. This has probably been a life-long pattern for them, and their response represents a continuity of their lifestyle, which is to be respected.

Large-Group Activities. Large-group activities generally require the least amount of interaction. For this reason, we might suggest that they are sometimes the least therapeutic. Paradoxically, they are the most frequent forms of activity, because they present the best image of the facility to visitors. They also often require the least amount of professional input; one person can run a film for 150 residents, or one caller can call out Bingo numbers for a roomful of people. Nonetheless, large-group activities are useful and necessary, as long as they are not the *only* available activities. In reality, people in the community play Bingo and go to the movies when they wish, but they also engage in other activities. The same choices should therefore be made available to those in a residential facility.

Large-group programs can be made exciting and special. Monthly birthday parties or entertainment by celebrities may encourage residents to dress up and prepare for a major event. These events also provide a very pleasant means of attracting families to visit with the residents. Also, the value of the use of community people to provide entertainment must not be underestimated, because it is most important that residents maintain a link with the outside world. Among the most common large-group activities are birthday parties, special holiday meals, entertaining films, musical programs, and (you guessed it) Bingo.

Religious Activities. Although it is debatable whether or not religious interest increases as one gets older, such activities must be provided, not only because of Medicare and Medicaid regulations, but also because (again) there must be a continuity of lifestyle.[8] Regular religious services should be offered, and clergy should be encouraged to make individual visits on a regular basis. In some facilities, residents may wish to assist with services or even conduct them. For example, in one facility, a resident played the organ for the Protestant services. The kind and scope of religious activities should be governed by the resident population. There would probably be daily services in a church-sponsored facility and weekly services in a nonsectarian residence. Scheduling is governed by space limitations and by other institutional realities. Regardless of the setting, interested patients should be encouraged to practice their beliefs and rituals as they wish, both formally and informally.

Goals of Activity Therapy

A good activities program generally improves the quality of life within a residential-care setting. As stated previously, activities help patients to function at optimum levels and thus foster independence, a sense of identity and purpose, and the opportunity to make choices. A program is therapeutic if it helps patients toward these goals. Persuading residents to participate in programs not to their liking is more indicative of coercion and authoritarianism than of therapy.[9] Realistically, many of the activities are diversionary, but recreation is, and should be, primarily *fun*. Recreation is about the only service in a facility that cannot be precisely prescribed. Although current legislation requires physicians to order activities for residents in institutional settings, no one can say, "Give this patient 2 gm of recreation." But a physician could order that "increased socialization" be encouraged. The method by which these orders are implemented should be devised by the recreation therapist and his or her staff.

Criteria for Success

The success of a program in institutional settings is too often measured in terms of the numbers attending. Although indications of success may sometimes be measured in terms of the numbers attending, this criterion seems inadequate. This is true even in community settings, where (presumably) an individual has more choice. For instance, summer camp programs for aging persons in the community may also be measured this way: the evening activity program is considered a failure or success strictly by a *count* of persons, not by the *meaning* of the experience to those people attending.

The general atmosphere of the nursing home, and the morale of the residents, may be more effective measures for judging the success of programs. Is the program offering residents opportunities for satisfactory experiences? Observation of such factors as interest, involvement, frequency of participation, enjoyment, growth, and socialization would provide clues for assessing this.[10]

Time and Frequency

Activities should be available during as many working hours as possible *every day* of the week. That residents "want" to go to bed early is a myth and generally reflects the fact that there is nothing for them to do in the evenings. Similarly, the often-heard statement that there should not be activities during visiting hours is indicative of the staff's attitudes rather than the residents' wishes. Obviously, scheduling activities must take institutional realities into account. For example, activities should not be scheduled until enough time has elapsed after breakfast for morning care, medications, and the like to be taken care of. Activities should not be scheduled in a room that is being used for other purposes, such as team conferences or in-service programs. It may be desirable, however, to schedule an activity during a mealtime, especially a picnic or an ethnic celebration. Conflicts with other therapies, such as physical or speech therapy, are generally best resolved between patients and therapists. If a patient likes "current events" discussion and it is only scheduled at 10:00 A.M., the physical therapist could perhaps schedule him or her at another time that day. Ideally, each staff member should be aware of a resident's complete daily schedule through some sort of charting device.

How much or how often a resident participates in activities is highly individual and depends to a great extent on interest and motivation. If the resident appears apathetic and if a professional feels that a particular activity may be "good" for such a resident, there might be a temptation for the professional to push her or him into that activity without asking whether or not the resident would enjoy it. Here, the professional is acting in an authoritarian way, and it is questionable how beneficial that activity will be to the client. It is often asked whether gentle coaxing is helpful if the team or the professional worker strongly feels that the client needs the recreation being offered. This is a difficult question. The answer must come from the institution's team, and there should be maximum input from the resident whenever possible. *Coaxing* is different from *pushing*, however!

A Written Schedule

A written schedule of activities should be prepared on either a weekly or a monthly basis. A few large, attractive, poster-sized schedules should be prepared for posting on bulletin boards and in other strategic places, such as the dining room or the front lobby. In addition, individual copies of the schedule should be distributed to each resident and to administration and other department heads. If the program is extensive, and if the budget and staff warrant it, monthly program booklets may be prepared. The activities worker may post the individual schedules in a strategic place—near the mirror or on the closet door—for slightly confused residents. Although the posted schedules should be attractive, they should be uncomplicated and highly legible. It is also a good idea to send annotated schedules to other department heads, with requests for assistance—to the dietary department with a request for refreshments for the birthday party or picnic, for example.

The Activities Leader

Many residential-care facilities have only one staff member who is responsible for activities. In reality, this person more often serves as a coordinator than as an activities leader. He or she does *not* conduct every activity and therefore does not have to be a "jack-of-all-trades." Instead, such a person is responsible for devising and implementing the activities schedule. Obviously, such a person must be familiar with the resources in the community. The more skillful a coordinator is in securing volunteer help, the more diversified the program will be. He or she must conduct many of the regularly scheduled programs, such as the birthday parties, the residents' council, card and game tournaments, and various crafts programs. An activities coordinator should be warm, empathic, well-organized, flexible, and able to integrate and implement new ideas.

Today there is a tendency toward more regulation and professionalism. Larger nursing homes have a registered recreation therapist as director of activities. Smaller facilities have a less trained person who works with a qualified consultant, who is a registered recreation therapist or registered occupational therapist.

Charting Progress

Besides planning and implementing the activities schedule, the activities coordinator is responsible for keeping records on patient activities. Initially the coordinator must put into the chart a record of an interview that reveals the patient's interests, hobbies, skills, and previous leisure experiences, as well as expressed interest in the facility's activities. Ongoing records must be kept of the patient's attendance, and into each chart, a monthly or quarterly summary of progress should be included. Progress notes should mention the patient's participation (or lack of it), changes in condition, successes or failures, and any modification of goals.

Of primary importance is the activities coordinator's ability to organize and transmit this information accurately and concisely. Since, at this time, there is no objective measure of activities programming, assessment depends on the activities leader's observations. Volunteers and co-leaders should be encouraged to report a patient's responses to the activities coordinator regularly. The coordinator should, of course, integrate this material into the chart notes.

MILIEU THERAPY

In milieu therapy, the total environment is used as a therapeutic modality. The patient designs his or her own therapeutic program, structuring the environment so that it most closely resembles the kind of setting that the patient was used to in the outside environment. This encourages patients to sustain social roles used in the outside community and also places responsibility for the roles and for environmental structuring on the patients themselves. A "structured series of meaningful behavioral expectations are formulated by both staff and patient, and positive reinforcement for appropriate behavior is emphasized." Patients in this type of program are grouped homogeneously, according to their primary needs, degree of independence and extent of disability.[11]

SUPPORTIVE GROUP PSYCHOTHERAPY

The history of group therapy or *group*, as it is informally known, includes rapid, dramatic change. As recently as 25 years ago, this approach was one of many for dealing with unhappy or unfulfilled people. It has since blossomed into a major social intervention, from traditional group therapy to the plethora of groups that exist today: encounter groups, human-potential groups, sensitivity-training groups, marathons, and leaderless groups.[12]

It has been found that, in dealing with the aging, the most suitable approaches are the supportive ones that emphasize resocialization of the person and a recognition of the need for promoting interdependence in the group, with increased self-sufficiency and potential for happiness. The traditional psychoanalytic group therapies attempt to deal with unconscious defense mechanisms, such as motivations, fantasies, and resistances.

Despite the rapid advances of group, psychotherapy—as a group experience involving older people—has never been readily available to the aged. Since therapy demands so much time and effort, it has been considered better to expend them on those who have a long life ahead.[13] This may be partly a result of the influence of Sigmund Freud, who suggested that psychoanalytic treatment was not particularly suitable for older people. Despite Freud's pessimism, however, other analysts attempted to use psychoanalytic approaches and have reported positive effects.[14] There has been a resulting change in the use of this therapy with the older adult; the attitude that intervention with the aging person is hopeless and that cure is almost impossible is undergoing a radical change.[15]

Goals in Supportive Group Approaches

The group approach is a psychological process in which a trained leader uses his or her particular skills to effect change in persons selected for the group. Group therapy has as its aim the promotion of better human relationships. For the aging group member, modified goals of treatment may be more realistic. Instead of focusing on personality reorganization, a more supportive approach would be to offer guidance as a means of catering to a patient's needs for assistance. In this approach, feelings of inferiority, acquired over a lifetime, are met with reassurance, and the patient's anxiety is relieved by the therapist, who assumes a protective role. The patient's guilt is also relieved by the therapist's permissive attitudes.[16]

A goal limitation is decided upon at the beginning of group treatment. No attempts to reawaken old conflicts should be made, since it is assumed that each member's group style reflects a lifestyle that has been used to derive gratification for her- or himself as a way of protection against injuries to self-esteem. Defense mechanisms are thus not tampered with.[17] The therapist here is a relatively active person who directs the course of therapy by providing guidance, reassurance, and environmental manipulation whenever necessary. The therapist tries to decrease anxiety in the patient and promote a feeling of being understood. Further, and most important, the client may be actively involved in solving his or her own problems. The therapist may also use some didactic measures, such as a discussion of what happens to the body as a result of aging, attitudes held by society toward the aging, ways of dealing with death, and other ideas. Therapist and client should be involved in an intense, satisfying interpersonal relationship. Sometimes this is the *only* relationship in the patient's current life. Supportive group therapy is, then, a means of attempting to re-establish an emotional balance that has been shaken by the many stresses of later years, not the least of which has been a move from the community setting to the institutional one. And even though its goals are limited, group therapy is known to have decreased older persons' fears and angers, improved their behavior and, in general, made for better overall functioning.

Target Population

Theoretically, any patient in a residential facility can be introduced to a group-therapy program after some preparation. In actuality, however, because of the limited number of trained people available, older residents selected for this approach are usually those who appear to be suffering from stresses with which they are unable to cope. For example, residents in one facility had to move from one floor to another. The authors observed that some patients seemed to manage very well but that others seemed to "fall apart," were more vulnerable. It is the latter patients who should be assigned to group therapy so that they can be helped to deal with the current stress. Similarly, people who have difficulty getting along with others, people who appear very depressed, anxious, agitated, or withdrawn, should also be assigned to group treatment.

Composition of the Group

Mixing personality types (heterogeneity) in group therapy appears to benefit the group. Participants may include depressed, suspicious, brain-damaged, or very regressed patients. If, for example, a group is made up of several depressed persons, it is often helpful to include some "starters" as part of the group—active, lively persons who act as catalytic agents to stimulate the entire group.

A group should generally consist of from eight to ten patients. If this is not feasible, there may be from six to eight. There should be enough group members to spur activity; if there are too few, there will be many "silent periods" and less spontaneity. Similarly, too many members will produce too much activity for both the leader and the group members. In addition, the more reticent patient may feel very lost in a large group.

Groups may be closed (the membership remains the same over a period of time) or open (the membership keeps changing). Once the group has been formed, other patients may ask to join. If possible, another group should be formed. If this is not possible, tact and patience should be used in explaining the exclusions. If it is possible that other groups will be formed in the future, interested residents should be told this, but *only* if this is a foreseeable reality; one should never raise false hopes.

Time

Although therapy groups may meet for an hour-and-a-half or two hours, the authors have found that groups of aging persons need less time, and a session can usually last from an hour to an hour-and-a-half without fatiguing its members. Sessions of less than an hour (e.g., 50 minutes) may also be helpful. The leader decides the time when the session will be held because he or she knows the daily schedules of other available activities. The group-therapy session should be scheduled at a time convenient to all.

Frequency

It is practical for a therapy group to meet once a week. Although more frequent sessions can be helpful, there is a shortage of personnel trained in this form of group therapy, and the pressures of their other duties and responsibilities must be considered.

Place

It is helpful to meet in a room that is attractive, well-lit, and comfortable, and where there will be as few disturbances as possible. The fewer distractions from the environment, the more energy can be devoted to the process taking place. In addition, the room should not be bare, because a bare room makes for a depressing atmosphere, and it should not be cluttered with objects, because clutter is distracting.

Chairs should be arranged in a rough circle, approximately less than one arm's length apart. There should be no table. Sitting around a table tends to dilute the group process, since members' bodies are partially hidden from view. A seating arrangement in which everyone is easily seen is preferred. The therapist sits within the circle, preferably toward a corner, because the diagonal position offers the best advantage for observing all patients at all times.

Materials

There are no special materials required for this group approach. It has sometimes been helpful to tape-record some of the sessions so that group members can play the tapes back for themselves. If the sessions are to be recorded, permission must be requested from all group members. Older persons are sometimes inhibited by the recording of the session. When permission has been sought and the goal explained—that is, for teaching/helpful purposes—recording of the session is often received with much enthusiasm by group members, many of whom have never had the opportunity to hear themselves on tape and are glad to have that chance now.

Written Schedule

A written schedule may be posted indicating the names of the patients in this program and the time, place, day, and date of the meeting. More often than not, however, the schedule is not posted because, despite the advanced thinking of our time, there is still some stigma attached to the words "group therapy," and patients may not wish to have their names posted. Usually, patients in a group-therapy program are aware of all of the details of the meetings and do not have to be reminded of them by having such information publicly displayed. Again, the nature of the patients, the facility, and the reality requirements are to be the determining factors.

The Leader

It is most important that the group-therapy leader have adequate training in conducting groups. Along with this, personal qualities of intuitive insight, the ability to be empathic, and an in-depth understanding of oneself are most helpful. The leader should not only be aware of his or her own self, feelings, ideas, attitudes, and perceptions, but should also be aware of every group member and should establish and maintain meaningful contact with each one. Since the leader plays a major role, he or she should sometimes offer instructional information but must beware of teaching too much. The leader should also have an optimistic attitude; when the group falters or seems unduly depressed, her or his optimism is often the most effective tool for rehabilitation. At times, such an attitude may be difficult to maintain, but its value cannot be overestimated.

A Therapy Session: Abbreviated Notes of a Recorded Session (Week Eleven)

Here is an abbreviated example of a group-therapy session conducted in a residential-care setting. The goal was to stimulate group interaction as a way of dealing with the members' expressed loneliness. In addition, support was given to group members' attempts to find solutions themselves as a way of bolstering their egos. The therapist allowed herself to be seen as a guiding person who could help them accept dependency feelings and who could encourage them to be independent. Memories were encouraged as a way of integrating past and present life. These expressed memories also provided clues to the therapist as to what resources the group member still possessed. These resources were then supported as a further means of strengthening the person's ego and ability to cope with current reality. Similarly, the therapist discussed the "outside" world (Washington, D.C.) as a way of linking the patient's former life to the current one.

Mrs. R.: It's good to be here for all reasons.

Therapist: What reasons?

Mrs. R.: Well, because otherwise, the week seems so long. It's a pleasure to come to talk to other people and to you, darling.

Mrs. C.: That's it. When I stay in my room here too long, sometimes I talk to myself. [*Laughs*.]
I talk to the walls too. Then I find something to do, like coming into the day room to watch TV. But how much TV can you watch?

Therapist: How about the others?

Mrs. B.: We come here to be with everyone—you, the nurse, everyone.

Mrs. K.: How was Washington? Did you tell the president about us? [*Everyone laughs. Reference is to a trip that the group leader recently made to Washington.*]

Therapist: [*Spends a few minutes telling of the trip to Washington and of some sights visited.*]

Mrs. C.: Washington is where everything happens. They have to know to make things better for older people.

Mrs. K.: But 30 or 40 years ago, we didn't even have this much. We just have to fight for things—then maybe you get some.

Therapist: What kinds of things in particular were you thinking of?

Mrs. C.: Well, poor people have to be helped.

Therapist: Could you spell that out . . . in what way?

Mrs. C.: Well, the poor are poor and the rich are rich. It could be better. But not only with money. Some people don't care for the poor people or the old people. It would take three hours to tell you.
[*Sighs.*]

Therapist: We don't have three hours, but we have some time, and I think maybe we can all discuss this. What do the rest of you think?

Mrs. C.: Mrs. R. can tell you.

Mrs. R.: I can tell you that now it's better. We never had Social Security. Now we have that and they even send somebody to clean your house if you need it, I am told. From this hospital, they sent a girl three times a week to the man who used to live next door to me, whose wife died. My daughter sees them and told me. They never used to do this.

Mrs. K.: If everybody pushes and fights, we'll get what we need.

Therapist: Good point.

Mrs. B.: Believe me, we all worked all our lives and we should get things from this country.

Therapist: Absolutely.

Mrs. K.: Will we be meeting some more?

Therapist: How do you feel about that . . . do you want to?

Mrs. K.: Sure. This helps. Coming to the group is good.

Therapist: In what way?

Mrs. K.: Well, in the group, we talk to each other, see each other more.

Therapist: You're saying you're lonely. What could you and all of us do about that?

Mrs. K.: We have to have more groups for us and even for some of the others, not just the one hour. That flies. The one hour is good but what is one hour? Last week, Mrs. R. (from another ward) came to sit in my room and talked to me for a while, and it was a real pleasure.

Mrs. R.: [*Laughs.*]
Then I invited her back. I wish I had some tea or something to give her, but she said she just wanted my company.

Therapist: I can understand that.

Mrs. H.: That's right. But we have to find things for us to do by ourselves—right, Doctor? We have to keep busy—otherwise the day is so long.

Therapist: Yes. A day can seem long if there is nothing to do. How about the rest of you . . . what do you think?

Mrs. C.: Right. We all have to help each other.

Mrs. K.: Back home . . . before here, I used to belong to clubs. That was the only thing that helped me . . . otherwise, you think too much. It used to help pass the time when my son couldn't come to see me often—when he moved away. We even had a community center in the building, and two evenings a week we used to go there and sing and tell stories. All the old people in the building used to go. It was nice.

Mrs. H.: We don't have a community center here—but we could get together by ourselves in the day room or someplace when the doctor is not here. We could just get together and talk to each other. The doctor said it was a good idea, right, Doctor?

Therapist: I think that's a fine idea. I would be glad to hear all about it. Try it for next time and let's talk about it in the group. See you next week.
[*States day and time.*]
So long until then.

QUESTIONS AND ANSWERS ABOUT SUPPORTIVE GROUP PSYCHOTHERAPY

What Are the Special Qualities, If Any, Of the "Good" Therapist? It has been said that the good therapist is an astute observer, a thoughtful listener, a tireless collector of data, a curious investigator, a disciplined clinician, and an independent thinker.[18] Although this may define the ideal therapist, the well-qualified therapist should have some combination of these characteristics.

What Happens When a Group Member Dies? This frequently happens in groups with the aged. When it does occur, the death should be discussed. The therapist can bring it up by saying something like "I heard that Mrs. G. died during the night," waiting for the group to respond. Exploration and in-depth discussions of the death should be attempted; such discussion should not be avoided.

What If a Group Member Says That He or She Does Not Want To Be In a Group With Another Group Member? This sometimes happens. Whenever possible, the suggestion should be made that it would be helpful for him, Mr. A., to stay in the group because talking about what bothers him about Mr. B. could be very important to him and to the others. If Mr. A. still refuses, he should be gently told that the group therapy sessions are voluntary and that he does not have to remain. If it is possible, he should be placed in another group.

How About Sex Distribution In Groups? Usually, there are many more females than males in these groups. If at all possible, a more equal distribution should be attempted, but if this is not feasible, it should help to have one or two men in a group with six women. The group in which the sexes are mixed has a very different quality from the group in which members are all of the same sex.

Doesn't Talking About Sex In a Group of Older People In an Institution Raise Problems About What to Do About It? Yes, but sex and sexual activity are natural aspects of life, and patients do have feelings about sex even when they do not talk about it. Discussing the subject in the group helps patients deal with these feelings. It is often an important area in which "life" can be brought back to the person.[19] How to resolve the issue of sexual activity between partners in the institution can also be discussed, and the group can be helped to find solutions to this problem.

When Are the Patients In a Group "Cured"? It all depends on the group and its members. Some members may be ready to leave a group before others are ready to leave. At that point, new members may be brought into the group. The "cure" has to do with the goals of the group and with the characteristics of the group and its members. There is no special time schedule for "cure."

Don't the Other Patients On the Ward Think Of the Person In Group Therapy As Being Crazy? That may be. The group-therapy program can help the person in the group to deal with this and with any pejorative attitudes expressed by others.

Do the People In the Group Become Closer To Each Other or More Hostile? This depends on the person and on his or her progress in the total group experience. Some people learn to feel closer to others in the group, but some feel more hostile. These feelings should be discussed by the group. Often people together in a group become good friends on the ward and develop a closeness that they had not shared before.

CHARTING PROGRESS

Almost all group therapists keep records or progress reports of sessions. Notes should not be taken during the session but, for the sake of accuracy, they should be written as soon after a session as possible. Notes are a way of keeping records of the group's progress and indicate to the therapist the direction in which the group is moving. These records should be shared with other staff personnel, because they provide information about group members that can greatly help staff in their planning activities with those patients. The group therapist should also make notes for her- or himself about the particular behavior of a group member in order to alert other staff that, for example, Mr. A. may be acting more depressed because of something that he is going through in the group. This alerts ward personnel not to be punitive but to understand that the depression is being dealt with in the group and that it may decrease over time.

REFERENCE NOTES

1. Meyer, H. D., & Brightbill, C. K. *Community recreation: A guide to its organization*, 3rd ed. Englewood Cliffs, N.J.: Prentice-Hall, 1964.
2. Haun, P. *Recreation: A medical viewpoint*. New York: Bureau of Publications, Teachers College, Columbia University, 1965, p. 39.
3. Donahue, W. Restoration & preservation of personality. In M. Leeds & H. Shore (Eds.), *Geriatric institutional management*. New York: G.P. Putnam's Sons, 1964, p. 180.
4. Avedon, E. M. Aging, apprehension and apathy. In H. Brantley & H. D. Sessoms (Eds.), *Recreation: issues and perspectives*. Columbia, S.C.: Wing Publications, Inc., 1969, p. 89.

5. Havighurst, R. J. The leisure activities of the middle aged. *American Journal of Sociology*, 1957, *63*, 152–162.
6. Covey, H. C. A reconceptualization of continuity theory: Some preliminary thoughts. *The Gerontologist*, December 1981, *21*(6), 628–633.
7. Bennett, R. (Ed.). *Aging, isolation, and resocialization*. New York: Van Nostrand Reinhold Co., 1980.
8. Blazer, D., & Palmore, E. Religion and aging in a longitudinal panel. *The Gerontologist*, 1976, *16*, 82–85.
9. Bennett, R. G., The meaning of institutional life. *The Gerontologist*, 1963, *3*, 64.
10. Weiner, M. B. The short-term effects of a resocialization program on the functioning of isolated, community-based geriatric clinic patients. In R. Bennett (Ed.), *Aging, isolation, and resocialization*. New York: Van Nostrand Reinhold Co., 1980, pp. 104–126.
11. Busse, E. W., & Blazer, D. M. *Handbook of geriatric psychiatry*, New York: Van Nostrand Reinhold Co., 1980, p. 321.
12. Rosenbaum, M., & Snadowsky, A. *The intensive group experience*. New York: The Free Press, 1976.
13. The old in the country of the young. *Time*, August 3, 1970, p. 50.
14. Grotjahn, M. Analytic psychotherapy with the elderly. *Psychoanalytic Review*, 1955, *42*, 419–427.
15. Weiner, M. B., & Wilensky, H. A psychotherapeutic approach to emotional problems of the elderly. *Journal of Nursing Care*, 1978, *11*(5), 14–15.
16. Goldfarb, A. I. Minor maladjustments of the aged. In S. Arieti & E. B. Brody (Eds.), *American handbook of psychiatry*, vol. 3. New York: Basic Books, 1974.
17. Weiner, M. B., & White, M. T. Self-psychology as an effective group approach with older adults. In: B. MacLennan, S. Saul, & M. B. Weiner (Eds.), *Group therapy in the mental health treatment of the elderly*. American Group Psychotherapy Assn. Monograph. New York: International Universities Press. (In press.)
18. White, M. T., & Weiner, M. B. *The practice of self-psychology*. New York: Brunner/Mazel, 1985.
19. Starr, B., & Weiner, M. B. *The Starr-Weiner report on sex and sexuality in the mature years*. New York: McGraw-Hill, 1982.

11

The Family As Part of the Therapeutic Team

While patients' groups in the residential facility may be new to them, each has been a member of a group, a family, all of his or her life. That first group was, and remains, the most important.[1] Emotional ties are made early and remain fairly constant. From early life on, a patient's style of living and way of handling all types of situations were learned in that group atmosphere. Think, for example, of how different families handle emotions such as anger: In one family, people may express anger through verbal confrontation and attempts at resolution. In other families, loud talking, shouting, or yelling may be the way in which annoyance or anger are expressed. In still other families, members may keep a lid on anger; indeed, may keep all strong feelings bottled inside themselves.

Patients, now in their later years, were influenced by these family styles from birth. At 4, 6, 12, and 16 years of age, they were responded to in certain ways in their families. By 60, 70, and 80 years or more, they have built up a lifetime of learned behaviors, and automatically respond in their own particular styles.

If patients have watched their parents keep emotions inside, chances are that they will do the same. Their learning ground, the family, was the only ball field in town; they had to play in it or not play at all. Now in a residential facility, they have a rich background of actions, behaviors, and responses that are very deeply a part of themselves. In a new environment, they will be repeating old behaviors while also learning new ones.

While about half of nursing-home residents are not close to their families, the other half has families who live nearby.[2] Placing the family member—mother, father, uncle, or aunt—in a nursing facility was no easy task. Despite the myth that Americans are uncaring, the record shows that, in fact, Americans do care, usually keeping their older kin at home for as long as possible.[3] When there is family, the older person lives with them until deeply troublesome behavior makes it impossible for the family to continue this care. A patient from a caring family will enter a nursing facility later in life than those who do not have families; elderly who lack caretakers move into nursing homes at younger ages.

The family who places the older adult in the care of others suffers a range of feelings. Along with anger, guilt, or sadness, there may also be relief. The care of an elderly parent may become a burden to family members who themselves are now middle-aged and are facing their own difficulties with aging. These feelings, with the complexities and conflicts that they present, may change continuously. The daughter, almost always the primary caretaker, may feel relief at the decision to place her parent in a nursing home—relief, however, accompanied by guilt and later anger, possible mixed with sadness.[4] Inevitably, many of these feelings will be displaced onto both the patient and the staff. The family member, in abdicating what she may feel is her family duty, now requires the nursing home to fulfill what had been her responsibility. The institution is, in this regard, the "parent" to the parent. As in all expectations of parents, only the "best" is accepted. That "best" represents what we have given, and would continue to give, to our parent. Anything less than that leaves us with guilt, frustration, and sadness.

A home in a community has had a familiar continuity, a background that has existed for many years. Everyone understands and knows each other's ways. The familiarity has been relaxing to us. The new home now offers many ambiguities. Ambiguity—uncertainty—makes us anxious.

Faced with chaos inside themselves and a strange, new environment outside, the family member feels as tense as a stranger in a foreign land. Discomforting questions may occur: what will this new place be like? Who will care for my parent? Who are all these professionals? How will I be able to clarify my parent's needs and get important messages about my parent across to these strangers? What will the future be like for my aging parent—and for myself? These questions deserve answers, and the family member seeks these answers as a way of allaying anxiety.

Professionals working with the older patient see the family member as a potentially helpful team person or as a hindrance to the team effort. Much depends on the initial interactions. As with many first impressions, these initial interactions make an impact. Since professionals already know the rules and workings of the environment with which they are dealing, one of the first tasks is to acquaint the concerned family person with the "rules of the game."

As consultants to nursing homes, the authors found most rewarding those weekend programs held for the convenience of families. These were designed to acquaint new families with the workings of the facility. Run for ten consecutive weeks, the sessions included appearances by representatives of all departments, who tried to familiarize families with the ways in which each department affected their loved one. "Recreation" spoke of who needed recreation, what the hours were, how results were measured, and, most important, who the contact person was for families seeking information. This focus was repeated by the other departments, including Nursing, Occupational Therapy, Physical Therapy, Dietary, Recreation, Psychiatry and Psychology, and Social Service. While different nursing homes may use different names for departments, and while states differ in regulations, most such facilities have several departments, interrelated and catering to the well-being of the aging patient. The family member needs to know who is in charge of whom, the conditions under which treatment takes place, and the focus of each department.

Of concern, too, are the facility's goals and expectations for the patient, and how departments cooperate to achieve that goal. For example, if the aging parent needs new eyeglasses, who will respond? Who will see to it? If arthritis has been a major complaint, which department will secure relief? Will this require occupational therapy, physical therapy, or drugs prescribed by the physician? Who is the person who will pass on such vital information to the family? When the family calls the nursing home, will they call a department, or the physician or nurse in charge? Will one become labeled as a "nuisance" to be avoided while seeking this information?

When family persons do not obtain information, ambiguity remains and anxiety increases. As tension within the person rises, so too does demand on staff. Staff, in turn, often retaliate with avoidance or brusqueness. The cycle then repeats itself, and relief becomes a far-fetched reality. The person hurt most in this scenario is the aging patient.

To intercede on behalf of the patient, the family and staff must join forces at the very beginning, when the older person first becomes a resident. The facility that can, at the onset, initiate a series of weekend meetings in which families—sometimes including three, four, or five concerned members—can meet to understand how that facility works can do much to ease future tensions. Sometimes, this means prolonging the life of the patient. For when family anxieties are eased, their interactions with the patient are relaxed and treatment has the best of chances.

Along with explaining the complexities of the nursing home to the family, the worker can also gain from family members an understanding of the lifestyle of the patient. While data may be scant on a patient's early history, any information gained is helpful. Early years are important, in that they are the formative ones, but the early or later middle years may also provide cues to individual lifestyles and ways of coping. Later years—the years before admission to the facility—also help tell the story.

A sensitive worker attempts to unravel the interweaving threads of the person's life. Every strand, examined for color, hue, texture, and weight, provides additional information, enabling the worker to form a picture of the patient. Together with the family, one can then plan the best of all schedules for the patient. What are his favorite hobbies? How would she feel about joining a particular group? How would he respond to occupational therapy? Would she do better in one-to-one situations or within a group? Should family members visit before or after a particular activity? What will make the patient the least anxious? The most anxious? What are his sensitive areas? What are her lifelong tastes and habits?

As the worker is gaining this needed information from family members, he or she is also observing the family, getting to know about their own styles of relating and living. The authors found weekends helpful for involving families (when families existed and were in any way interested), since many family members, including daughters and sons, work during the week and told us that only weekends were possible. If time can be arranged, an excellent way of providing relief for patients and families is to involve the family in a group situation.

The modalities that we have described, such as sensory training, reality orientation, remotivation, and other approaches, are for the impaired elderly and, as specialized techniques, can be led by a staff person trained in these techniques—psychologist, nurse, recreational therapist, aide or orderly. However, conducting groups for the community-living, well-functioning person of any age requires special group training. But its value should not be understated.

If a family member shows *any* interest in becoming a group participant, and if the facility has such trained persons willing to conduct such a group (either as a full-time staff person or as a hired consultant), the family member should be encouraged to join "group." Again, we emphasize that particular skills are necessary. Though groups for relatives of the impaired elderly are rare, they do exist. The professionals who conduct them are usually experienced practitioners, such as nurses, psychologists, psychiatrists, social workers, and others trained in "group."

CONDUCTING GROUPS WITH FAMILY MEMBERS

The focus of a group containing family members of institutionalized persons would be to help them deal with the strains and pressures they feel in relation to their older relatives. Such a group would offer some didactic information about the aging process itself—the symptomatic behaviors of organic brain syndrome and of genuine senility; the impact of drugs; how memory is affected by depression, aging, circulatory, and respiratory problems; and incontinence.

Along with these subjects, life-long development should become part of the group discussion. Family members can assess their own roles within the family and can understand any ambivalences that they may have, as well as the stresses and strains intrinsic to a move such as relocation to a nursing home, and can see how these factors interact with life-long personality characteristics.

The functioning of the nursing home as the "parent" to the family is also part of this group learning experience. As stated, since the group will become the "instrument for learning, helping, supporting, and problem solving," the worker needs skills in both group processes and teaching.[5]

As regards conducting groups for the elderly themselves, time and place are determined at the convenience of both group and staff members. It has been found that a closed group is more effective than an open one and that a set time sequence (such as eight sessions) is preferred to unlimited time. As is typical for groups, approximately six to ten members can be included and the sessions conducted for an hour-and-a-half once a week.

We have suggested that family members become involved with a group when some interest is shown. That interest is not always visible but may be there nonetheless. Couched in other words, interest is sometimes revealed through expressions of concern for the older relative or through complaining. The following is such an example:

[*A nurse clinician is speaking with a family member who has asked to see her in order to tell her something about the family member's father, a fairly new patient in the facility.*]

Mrs. A.: Thanks for making time for me. I'm really quite upset.

Nurse: I'm glad that I was able to see you, and I apologize for keeping you waiting a while. What seems to be the problem?

Mrs. A.: Well (pauses), it's my father, Mr. L. You know him, of course?

Nurse: Yes. He's fairly new here, but I do know him.

Mrs. A.: He's unhappy and complains (long pause) . . . about his room, his roommate, roaches in the dining room—a whole bunch of things. He wants to leave.

Nurse: What do you think about his wanting to leave?

Mrs. A.: Oh well, I don't think it's possible, in his condition. You see, he lived with me and my family until it became impossible for us to care for him.

Nurse: You know, in my experience, sometimes when a patient wants to leave and complains, he's really saying something other than just what seems to be expressed. That is not to say that complaints are never justified. But, do you think he's saying that he wants to come back home to live with you again? My own thinking is that this may be what he's feeling.

Mrs. A.: Now that you say it, I think that's so. I only know that, as he starts complaining about his room, for example, I start feeling so jumpy and edgy that I just want to get away, and then I feel guilty for wanting to leave him.

Nurse: I can understand your feelings. You both love him and want the best for him but, wanting the best, you feel that you can no longer take care of him at home; knowing his condition, I'm inclined to agree. It's a common problem. What could be helpful is for you to possibly talk about this with others in your situation. We are beginning a group here with family members of the patients. Would you be interested in joining? My sense of it is that it would work for you and make you feel better. We plan to meet for eight weeks on ______________ day at ______________ o'clock. Is that possible?

Mrs. A.: It makes my schedule a little tight, but I think I can make it. I'll give it a try because, feeling the way I do now, when I visit (long pause) is just not a very good feeling. I'll try anything that can make me feel better.

Nurse: Good. I'm glad you decided to give it a try. I think you'll find it most helpful.

An anticipated result for Mrs. A. and for other group members would be: some change in their behavior toward their elderly relative, change in their beliefs about aging itself, increased awareness of the facts of aging—biological, psychological, and social—and some insights into their relationships with their older relative, both in the current situation and over their entire lifespan.

INVOLVING THE PATIENT

It is important that, whenever possible, the patient should be involved in all of this planning. In the case of Mrs. A., for example, the patient should be told that his daughter is in a group conducted by the facility for family members. While the contents of the group discussions are private and are not shared with the patient, sharing the fact of his daughter's attendance indicates her desire to help him, along with helping herself. This can only benefit the patient by raising his self-esteem and increasing feelings that "she cares." If other feelings, such as "What does she need a group for?" intermingle with this, these should also be handled by staff and should not be ignored. In this way, family members, staff, and patient interlock, each unit interested in the others.

Working together, these three units thus act as a team. As in all teams, information should intersect, each of the units supplying what is necessary to ensure a tight, closely knit network. Aware of another's workings, the staff person now knows the family and its system as far back as its history is available. Information forms a cumulative body of knowledge, leading up to and including the recent decision for placement. The patient now knows both the routines of the facility and the answers to practical questions, including who is in charge of what department, what her or his daily routine will be like, and how family members can fit into this new schedule.

The third unit, the family, is now better acquainted with, and sensitive to, the new facility. With this familiarity, family members can now visualize how they and the patient fit into this new situation. Aware of the pecking order within and between departments, they are relieved to know that, should they feel anxious or wish further information, they can call and gain answers to their questions. As their knowledge increases, apprehension and anxiety decrease. Feeling at ease, they can then deal with the complexities of the new situation; chaos has given way to a sense of order and peace.

Time heals the wound that family members may feel in placing a loved one in an institution. Eventually, family members may direct all of their energies toward working to integrate the patient into the new environment. That will enable the patient to live whatever years are left with satisfaction, and even joy.

REFERENCE NOTES

1. Weiner, M. B., Teresi, J., & Streich, C. *Old people are a burden but not my parents*. Englewood Cliffs, N.J.: Prentice-Hall, 1983.
2. Ibid.
3. Ibid.
4. Ibid.
5. Hartford, M. E., & Parsons, R. Use of groups with relatives of dependent older adults. In S. Saul (Ed.), *Group work with the frail elderly*. New York: The Haworth Press, 1983, p. 80.

PART III

The Community Aged

12

The Community Aged

The vast majority of the aged do not live in institutions; they remain in the community. A significant proportion of this large group of older people remains very active, sometimes through participation in senior-center activities. The community aged also become involved in church and church-related programs, remain employed as part-time workers, or are increasingly interested in continuing their education at various schools and colleges. Still others retain a strong family orientation by fulfilling grandparent (and other) roles.

Many of the community elderly can be observed sitting in parks and in other places where people gather. This 95 percent of the aged population is extremely varied, their needs and situations very individualized, and their problems and strengths very specific. The vast majority of this group might be called the *active aged*, in the sense that they comprise individuals who are physically healthy and fairly mobile. In contrast, the remaining proportion of the community aged could be termed the *passive aged*, in the sense that they are less ambulatory, perhaps in poorer health, but do not reside in an institution.

The active aged comprise the majority of what is increasingly being termed the *young–old*. The young–old are people between the ages of 55 and 75 who are distinguished as a group by the common fact of having experienced retirement. The young–old currently make up approximately 15 percent of the United States population. This age group is viewed by many social scientists as becoming ever more educated, increasingly concerned with self-development, psychologically and physically vigorous, and interested in discovering meaningful uses for their leisure time. It is expected that those who work with the community aged will be dealing more and more with the needs, hopes, and aspirations of such people.

The passive aged will soon comprise the majority of what has recently been termed the *old–old*. The old–old, or those people 75 and over, often continue to live in the community but become increasingly dependent on supportive social services and prosthetically designed physical environments. Although we have made some distinctions between the active aged and the passive aged and between the young–old and the old–old, we can still talk about some general problems faced by the community aged as a group.[1]

PROBLEMS OF THE COMMUNITY AGED

The problems faced by the community aged might be described in terms of the following problem source areas: economic, physical, social, psychological, and philosophical. Each source area poses significant conflicts and stresses with which older people often have to cope. In fact, it is proposed that the goals of any comprehensive rehabilitation or service program could only be truly achieved by helping the elderly deal with all of these problem source areas successfully. Unfortunately, most programs seem to focus on only a few of these source areas at any one time; few seem to be equipped to assess and serve the full spectrum of needs. Following is an outline of these problem source areas and the stresses that they induce.

Problem Source Area	Related Stress
Economic	Adjusting to income loss and to a new lifestyle upon retirement.
Physical	Adjusting to the experience of body changes, some health deterioration, decreased mobility, and decreases in sensory capacities.
Social	Adjusting to potential loss of social status, lack of adequate replacements for social roles, and the need to evaluate leisure needs as independent of work needs.
Psychological	Adjusting to the realization of no longer being young and the resultant feelings about the self. New developmental tasks and crises become important, while old issues (such as *Who am I?*) re-emerge and become newly central.
Philosophical	Coming to grips with existential and/or religious issues. The issues of *Why am I? What is my life about? What is life in general about?* come into the foreground of thought.

Although people of all ages must deal with these issues, they are more salient as a group of problems for the aged. That is, the aged are often in the position of having to experience—and cope with—all of the above problems simultaneously. In contrast, younger people usually must resolve issues related to only one or two problem source areas at a time and, when stress experiences do occur, they are not as acute as they are for the aged.[2]

TANGIBLE APPROACHES IN THE COUNSELING MODE

The methods and techniques of working with older people must inevitably differ from approaches used with younger people. In particular, counseling older people should focus on tangible interactions, as opposed to purely interpersonal sensitivity-group approaches. In other words, the counselor should use a topic—something tangible—as an environmental prop through which to relate. This general guideline has a number of advantages: First, it decreases anxiety among participants. Second, it creates a focus for counseling that is quickly understood by participants. Third, it provides options for the counselor, such as staying at content (superficial) information-exchange levels, as opposed to going into personal (in-depth) feeling levels.[3]

Something tangible is characterized by qualities that are immediately perceivable. Tangible counseling approaches usually involve clear goals and purposes, such as teaching skills, developing interests, or discussing topics. Structured, time-limited, problem-centered group approaches might be considered tangible because they provide external material through which people relate. The senior center that provides time for specific classes, training in specific skills, or discussion groups around specific topics might thus engender greater group and individual participation than a center that provides more abstract general counseling or therapy. This latter approach, although useful, might be more emotionally threatening or might not be as easily understood by the elderly living in the community and is better reserved for those who specifically seek psychotherapy.

A number of group-based counseling intervention approaches have emerged that seem to deal with the problems engendered by the social, psychological, and philosophical problem source areas that we have mentioned. One such approach, *life enrichment counseling*, an approach that stresses peer counseling, will be presented here.[4,5]

LIFE ENRICHMENT

Any person's life history is a recording of his or her attempts to add positive experiences. Such experiences are the "nutrients" necessary for an enriched life. It is only under certain conditions, such as increased stress, that this tendency toward life enrichment appears to wane, becomes inhibited, or is arrested altogether. The person whose main source of enrichment came from the work role but who is forced to retire may feel dysfunctional. He or she may be unable or unwilling to add new, positive experiences to life. What is experienced as positive may depend to a great extent on cultural values, internalized social norms, and personality characteristics.[6] Many older people who experience stress as a function of the various problem source areas may therefore have inhibited their tendency toward life enrichment. From this point of view, counseling, or working with, the aged involves developing methods and approaches to reawaken the tendency toward self-enrichment.

Characteristics of the Enriched Person

If we are to work toward the development of any goal, it is helpful to be guided by some criteria for defining the enriched person. The enriched individual adds positive experiences by:

1. Successfully resolving developmental crises and tasks as they emerge.
2. Constructing her or his life (passivity is not the principle mode of relating to the world).
3. Functioning as an open system: he or she seeks new information and considers new ideas.
4. Continuing to make an impact on others.
5. Becoming involved in activities considered subjectively meaningful.
6. Developing a differentiated ego structure linked to a consistent core self.
7. Maintaining a sense of spontaneity instead of being driven by impulsive actions.
8. Keeping a sense of humor that can be shared with others.

The above criteria are meant as guidelines, not as an all-inclusive list. We shall now further explain their meaning.

Successfully Resolving Developmental Crises and Tasks As They Emerge. Following Erickson's, and other, developmental theories, we note that the personality-shaping experiences with which people are confronted keep changing throughout the life span. Many of these experiences are, in fact, not age-related but situation-related, and thus may repeat themselves at various points in the life cycle. For example, according to Erikson, the older person who, upon reviewing his or her life, feels that it has generally been worthwhile may be successfully resolving the developmental crisis of integrity versus despair but may also be faced with the recurring crisis of intimacy versus isolation because of the death of a spouse or the loss of good friends.

Constructing One's Life. The construction analogy implies a sense of building upon a foundation that is continuously elaborated upon as life goes on. This is not the same as the maturational concept of "growth," which implies a natural, uninfluenced development. The construction analogy implies that the person needs to feel some involvement in, and responsibility for, her or his own growth (that is, in part, the person constructs his or her life). Working with the aged often involves helping people re-experience this feeling. Presumably, people who continue to experience life in this manner will feel a combined sense of growth, development, and change—in short, that they are enriching their own lives.

Functioning As an Open System. An open system denotes the ability to acquire, and be influenced by, new information. Individuals who function as open systems have the opportunity to continue enriching their lives with those nutrients that add to their growth and development. That is, they seek and consider new information about themselves and their relation to the world. Without this ability, people cannot change, and thus, the possibility of growth and development is stopped. A closed system is a system that does not accept new information. It is as if there were a permanent barrier preventing new information from entering (Fig. 12–1). Those who function as closed systems may be thought of as living in another cultural period or historical era, as if they need to maintain the world outlook that characterized life at an earlier age.

One example of a closed system was described by an acquaintance who told the story of his aged aunt, who supported him through college. Upon his graduation, she strongly tried to influence him to take a job in a "safe" civil-service profession instead of going into the computer-programming field, which was then (the early 1960s) a relatively new profession. The reason for her feelings was that she vividly recalled the depression of the 1930s and remembered how, although most people in business lost their jobs, those in the civil service were relatively secure. This set of values may have been relevant in the 1930s but was no longer so in light of the relative affluence of the 1960s (nor was it relevant in the 1970s, for that matter, with the increased layoffs experienced in the formerly secure civil-service occupations). It seemed to this young man that his aunt had not allowed new information (in the area of business) to "enter in" since the depression and that she had retained a depression-era psychology.

Continuing To Make an Impact On Others. This notion implies that, ultimately, we are social beings and that we need a sense of relationship with others in order to feel that our lives are being enriched. The quality of the relationship may be very important. A social relationship (such as playing checkers) may be pleasant, but it

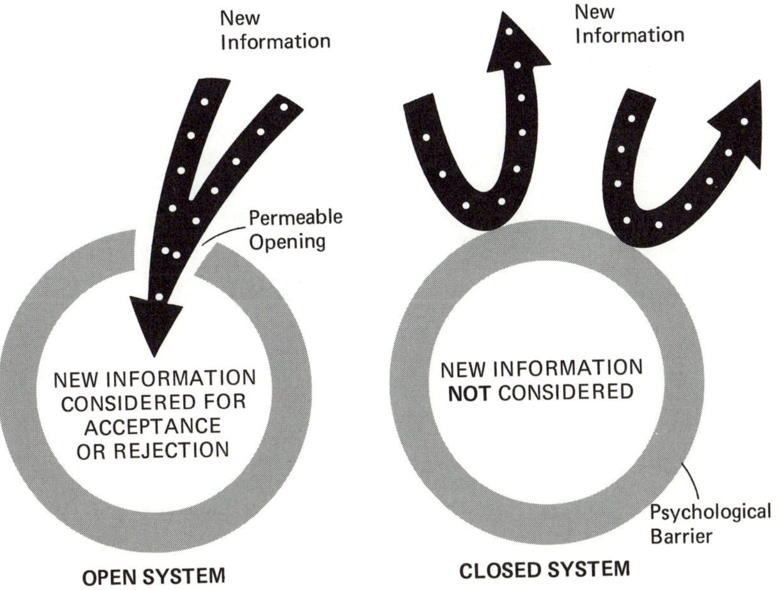

Figure 12–1. Open and closed life systems.

does not necessarily lead to a sense of enrichment. One important qualitative aspect is implied by the term *impact*, which connotes the sense of experiencing oneself as making an impression that is clearly perceived in terms of the reaction of some other to one's thoughts, feelings, or actions. The term impact, as used here, is neutral. That is, another's reaction to what we say, do, or think may be either positive, negative, or merely acknowledged in some clear way.

The crucial aspect is that what we say, do, or think is given some import: the other person responds as an open system to our encounter. When this occurs, we feel that we have entered into another's area of experience. Such a feeling may provide a sense of well-being. This situation, of course, should work reciprocally. The enriched person thus feels that she or he is part of the social community if her or his words, thoughts, and actions are given due consideration (whether they are agreed with or disagreed with). It is only when we are ignored or when we ignore others that we begin to feel isolated and alienated; such experiences can provide avenues for various forms of psychological retreat and withdrawal.[7]

We are suggesting, then, that the feeling of physical isolation sometimes felt by older people is exacerbated by the experience of interpersonal isolation to which it is related. One of the nutrients that enriches an older person's life is the experience of interpersonal validation of that person's experiences. Without this social sense of impact, we do not feel completely human. There is some experimental evidence to support this point of view. Work in sensory deprivation, for example, indicates that prolonged periods of physical and interpersonal isolation can lead to a sense of ego disintegration.[8]

To some extent, such experiments might be prototypical of what is experienced by the aged when important aspects of their interpersonal environment are removed—for example, the death of valued friends or the loss of valuable social experiences gained through work. These experiences appear to encourage the process of disengagement, or withdrawal, from society. Psychologists have noted that one of the most difficult tasks with which older people have to deal is the loss of feeling validated and worthwhile in the eyes of others who are significant in their lives, such as friends, family, and work associates.[9] In terms of the problem source areas previously mentioned, it seems that *who* we are, *why* we are, and *how* we feel about our social roles and status very much depend on the reciprocal impact that we have on those around us. Working with the aged implies encouraging them to enter into situations that promote the possibility of reciprocal impact.

Becoming Involved In Activities Considered Subjectively Meaningful. In working with people of any age, an important task is to help them to discover hidden resources or to actualize latent potentials. For the community aged, the issue of worthwhile use of leisure time may emerge as an important problem. Frantically engaging in any activity in order to prevent boredom or to avoid feelings of anxiety often tends to be ultimately unsatisfying. Yet, many people (including the community aged) seek fulfillment by such means.

Understanding just what is worthwhile or satisfying is a very complex topic that many psychology writers have avoided.[10] We believe that this understanding must always come from within, from the subjective experience of the person. For our purposes, we shall consider that any worthwhile activity must do the following:

- Involve free choice.
- Often demand some effort.
- Be felt as intrinsically rewarding.
- Perhaps aid toward the resolution of a developmental task.

We might note that the above criteria can apply to any activity, whether work or leisure.[11] It is when these criteria are not consistently met by our activities that we may begin to experience life as meaningless. The individual who engages in activities merely to please others or out of a sense of conformity may be missing important enrichment nutrients. Working with the community aged implies developing methods to help people to experience meaning in significant portions of their lives.

Developing a Differentiated Ego Structure Linked To a Consistent Core Self. The term differentiated ego structure refers to the many different life roles through which we gain a sense of social identity and through which we validate a sense of personal identity. These roles and activities may be those of a husband, wife, truck driver, teacher, student, religious observer, and so on. No one of them fully defines who we are, but each reflects one aspect of ourselves. Although, to some extent, our style of involvement in our various roles is a function of cultural expectations, it is also a reflection of our core self.

As an analogy, we might note that a famous artist might paint, sculpt, draw, or design textile patterns, working with various media. Although each medium looks different, somehow all of the artist's productions are recognized as a product of his or her self. A Picasso is thus recognized as such, no matter what medium the work is in. If we conceive of social roles as the media of life, then we may suppose that all of them are affected by our basic, core self; however, none can completely reflect this self.

Each role is linked to the self. Problems arise, however, when the role and the self are not linked together. The individual who overidentifies with the role of the worker, as if it were not linked to a core self but *was* the core self, will have a terrible crisis when that role is lost through retirement.

The enriched person, then, realizes that the most that one can do is to lend oneself to a role but that one can never totally become the role (although one may better develop oneself through being in that role). This notion is especially important for the aged, since they are particularly subject to role loss. From this point of view, the ingredients that enrich the lives of old people consist of new ways of experiencing and differentiating their ego structure, through which to express the basic, core self. Expression of the core self can occur through new leisure, work, family, or community experiences.

Maintaining a Sense Of Spontaneity. Spontaneity should be distinguished from impulsiveness. Although both impulsive and spontaneous acts are characterized by little thought, they are distinguishable in terms of how they are experienced. An impulsive activity has a "driven" quality: one feels that the impulse *must* be acted upon. If it is not acted upon, there is a strong sense of frustration or discomfort.

Impulses meet certain unsatisfied needs that may be either conscious or unconscious. A spontaneous act is experienced as the product of free choice, in that people feel free to either act or not act upon their choices. There is no sense of conflict within them; there is no blockage. If they choose not to act, there is no strong sense of frustration. They feel ready but do not have to do any particular thing. The tendency toward spontaneity seems to depend on feeling comfortable and secure in one's social and psychological world. As people age, they may lose their sense of spontaneity. We suggest that it is important to maintain this sense of spontaneity and that those who work with the aged should find ways to reawaken this feeling. This might be accomplished through leisure or other forms of group counseling.

Keeping a Sense Of Humor That Can Be Shared With Others. The ability to laugh at oneself and with others is perhaps a unique human ability. Humor helps relieve the seriousness of life and provides a validation that both the world and the self are to be enjoyed. By humor, we do not mean cynical, self-deprecating humor or the humor of denial. We mean the ability to accept the world as being other than only a serious place and about being able to validate this feeling with peers. Two important basic abilities involved in our meaning of humor are the ability to appreciate or laugh at someone else's humor and the ability to self-generate humor (such as telling jokes). Most people seem to have fully developed the first ability, but the second is sometimes more difficult for people to develop.

In sum, humor is important because it adds to the joy of life and to feelings of well-being. Working with the community aged should mean going beyond helping them deal with only serious life tasks. It may be equally as crucial to help them to develop a sense of humor.

THE LIFE-ENRICHMENT COUNSELING APPROACH

The life-enrichment counseling approach is a structured counseling module.[12] Through a guided discussion format that uses structured materials, it focuses on how to help recognize problems and develop approaches so as to make the best use of leisure time. The goal is to help assess and develop the creative, satisfactory use of time for people at different life stages. By development, we are often speaking in terms of relevant psychosocial issues, such as how do we help the community aged gain a sense of identity, generativity, or integrity through use of their leisure?

The guiding philosophy of the life-enrichment approach is proactive instead of purely rehabilitative, in the sense that it is aimed at helping to enhance persons' developmental potential. It is also rehabilitative, in that it aims to restore a person's capacities for experiencing a sense of growth and to reinstate feelings of worth through group interaction with peers.

Format

Although the format is flexible, life-enrichment counseling essentially involves the following sequence of eight possible phases:

1. Introduction of the module.
2. Self-generated list of leisure activities.
3. Self-evaluation of enjoyment.
4. Assessment of developmental experiences through leisure.
5. Ecological assessment of activities.
6. Qualitative descriptions.
7. Theme-oriented discussion.
8. Individual counseling or follow-up.

At times, phases are added or deleted for certain populations. Phases other than introduction of the module and self-generation of leisure activities are independent and do not have to follow in any particular sequence. For illustration purposes, we shall discuss the use of this module with a target group of community aged; for example, senior-citizen-center participants.

Phase 1. Introduction of the Module. The rationale for introducing the module to participants can vary, depending upon the setting and the purpose involved. As part of a senior-center program, the module may be introduced as a potentially diverting activity involving the discussion and exchange of ideas about how leisure time can be used, with the group leader acting as moderator. The module can also be introduced as a discussion of the philosophical issues of leisure from religious or other points of view. In more clinical settings, it might be used as a structured projective method for discussing in-depth feelings about the self. Use of the module ultimately depends on the purpose of the group and the skill of the leader. It is important that all leaders be aware that they are dealing with what can rapidly become sensitive topic areas.

Phase 2. Self-Generated List of Leisure Activities. Upon introduction, participants are presented with the first of three evaluation forms: Self-Generation of Leisure Activities (see Appendix E). Each participant is asked to make a list of the things that she or he does during leisure time. There are no constraining present categories, such as checklists. Participants are encouraged to make their lists as long as they wish, although it is sometimes useful to have a minimal time limit (say ten minutes). This allows each person enough time to complete his or her list. Creativity theory has suggested that initial-thought associations to a word or concept tend to be normative or stereotyped and that, with time, more unusual and creative responses may emerge.[13] This is especially true for individuals whose anxiety levels are high. Older people who might be more subject to internal and external stresses may need more time to get to truly personal interests.

Very frequently, participants will ask, "What is work and what is leisure?" It is often useful to defer this question until later discussion and let the participants decide the issue for themselves. We suggest telling participants to list whatever meets their own criteria for leisure. For example, many people put down such things as housework, which some might consider a nonleisure activity. Nevertheless, housework may legitimately be experienced as leisure by certain people. This approach is in keeping with the concept of life enrichment; that is, that people need to construct their lives and to subjectively determine the meaning of their own activities.

If participants are the community aged (such as the young–old), the evaluation form can be self-administered. If participants are the more impaired, the directions can be read to each person, and another member of the group (or the group leader) can write down the participant's responses.

Phase 3. Self-Evaluation of Enjoyment. After describing the various ways in which leisure time is used, participants can be asked to evaluate the degree of enjoyment that they experience when involved in each activity. Each person does this by circling the number that best expresses his or her degree of enjoyment for each activity recorded in the self-generated list. The numbers to be circled are printed in the *Degree of Enjoyment* portion of the Self-Generation of Leisure Activities form. These numbers range from 1 through 5, where 1 stands for "little enjoyment" and 5 stands for "much enjoyment."

This exercise can provide a general picture of how people feel about the kinds of activities that they subjectively list as part of leisure time. It can provide an opportunity for discussion about specific activities that are enjoyed. This discussion also allows each participant to discover similar interests and enjoyments in others, thereby providing the opportunity for validating feelings of self-esteem and self-worth.

Phase 4. Assessment of Developmental Experiences Through Leisure. After participants have completed their lists and their enjoyment ratings, they are presented with a list of developmental-task descriptors (see Activity Gains in Appendix F). These descriptors consist of eight phrases that describe developmental stages.[14] Each respondent is asked to indicate which phrase best expresses what might be gained from each activity listed during the self-generation phase. Theoretically, the exercise should provide the developmental meaning of each person's activity repertoire. Gains are to be listed by number on the right-hand side of the first form (Self-Generation of Leisure Activities).

Provisions can be made for respondents to indicate more than one descriptor for each activity listed. Participants can be asked to list (under the gains column in the first form) the numbers of as many descriptors as they feel apply to each leisure activity. Respondents are not required to provide descriptors for activities that do not seem to meet any of their developmental needs, as described in the second form (Activity Gains). The descriptors used here are illustrative phrases. It should be clear that other descriptors may be substituted, depending on the situation and population. The descriptor approach is useful for purposes of subsequent discussion, rather than for assessment. (The descriptors can be read to participants who find it difficult to read or write.)

Phase 5. Ecological Assessment of Activities. This task involves the presentation of the third form, Radius of Activities (see Appendix G). Participants are asked to look over their Self-Generation of Leisure Activities form and to think of the locations in which each of the listed activities is normally carried out. They are then asked to refer to the list of eight "locales" provided in the third form and to enter the appropriate number in the "place" column provided in the first form. Participant responses may indicate the extent of the exploratory activities of each person. The participant responses can also be used for subsequent discussions about concepts of "neighborhood" and to encourage exploratory activity.

Phase 6. Qualitative Descriptions. This task requires that each participant describe what he or she experiences in (or from) the activities engaged in. These qualitative descriptions should be written or listed in the activity-gains column of the first form. This phase leads to Phase 7, the theme-oriented group discussion.

Before we turn to Phase 7, we must note that the first six phases are presented as guidelines. It has been our experience that they do not have to be followed rigidly. In many cases, only some of the phases may be relevant. Indeed, each phase may be carried out as a separate unit over a period of days or weeks. Their appropriateness depends on the kind of group and on time allowances.

Phase 7. Theme-Oriented Group Discussion. By theme-oriented group discussion, we mean a situation in which participants are encouraged to focus on themes or issues of common concern and interest. The theme-oriented group is especially useful for the beginning worker (or counselor), because the focus remains on a tangible topic. As previously suggested, one such topic might be various uses of leisure time. Since it is not necessary to spend a great deal of time focusing on the analyses of emotional relations within such a group, the beginning counselor is free to focus on creating an atmosphere of mutual participation and trust, through which a sense of group cohesiveness may develop. The more experienced worker will find ample material for opening up emotionally laden areas if this seems appropriate or if the participants expect such discussion. The tangible-theme group thus provides flexibility for various counseling or educational needs.

A theme-oriented group is less stressful for aged populations because its structure provides the opportunity to share feelings and ideas about specific topics of mutual interest. For example, by virtue of each person's involvement in the series of exercises and discussions about the uses of leisure time, a sense of "connectedness" among the participants is potentially established. In general, sharing common interests provides a "launching pad" for deeper discussion.

Following are some suggestions for guiding a theme-oriented group in terms of the six phases previously discussed. Have the participants arrange themselves in small groups (of six or seven) by sitting in a circle or around tables.

Uses For the Self-Generated Leisure Activities Form. The material generated by the participants provides the basic discussion resource for the worker or counselor.

The simplest discussion technique requires asking each participant to read out loud the items that he or she has written. This exercise encourages participants to reveal something personal and subjectively meaningful about themselves that can be shared with others. It encourages participants to see similarities between themselves and others, and it enhances a sense of "connectedness" and group cohesion. As a result, an open, theme-oriented discussion can ensue about the variety of activities that people engage in. Such a discussion can serve as an icebreaker for a newly formed group in a senior-citizen or other community center. Although it does reveal material that is personal, it also allows people the choice of not becoming involved in any underlying emotional content if they do not want to. (Participants do not have to read every item on their lists if they choose not to.)

Material produced by the self-generated lists can also be used to develop a more philosophical or more topical discussion about the use of time. In this approach, the worker's aim is to suggest that participants discuss "what is defined as leisure and what is not." The attempt to clarify differences between work and leisure is not always simple and can often lead participants into a stimulating discussion about the meanings given to various life activities. The discussion may also help participants to understand the subjective element in each one's personal value system. This, in turn, can encourage the appreciation of differences between oneself and others.

One method for implementing these aims is to ask participants to read their lists out loud (this should be on a voluntary basis) and then discuss whether or not they agree on what is work and what is leisure. For example, the leader might ask: "Do some of you consider what anyone else describes as leisure to be work? Why? Did anyone not include what Mr. Jones put down because you thought of it as work? How many people put down 'cleaning house' as a leisure activity? Is it leisure for some and work for others? Why? How did each of you go about defining what was a leisure activity? Should we all go by the same set of definitions?"

We have also noted that some people characteristically omit, or prefer not to immediately discuss, certain items. For example, some people leave out sex as a leisure activity. With some humor, we have sometimes suggested that this might mean that it is considered work! In a more serious vein, focusing on the issue of sex can lead to fruitful clinical counseling discussions about an area of human functioning that is very sensitive to many older people.[15] It has happened that people who are embarrassed about having sexual needs and interests at an "inappropriate age" find it both easier and less anxiety-provoking to change or discuss their attitudes upon discovering that others in the group find sex to be an appropriate topic that can be talked about. Thus, both the exchange of self-generated leisure items among participants and the discussion of what are and what are not leisure activities can yield a number of important social learning experiences. This, in turn, may help clarify such questions as "Who am I?" (psychological), "Why am I?" (philosophical), and feelings about social status. When others approve of one's ideas and activities, or at least suggest that they are worthy of discussion, good feelings about the self may follow.

Uses For the Self-Evaluation Of Enjoyment Rating Form. The simplest use for the enjoyment-rating material involves a slight modification of the technique described for use of the self-generated activity lists. This modification requires that each participant (on a voluntary basis) read out loud the activities that he or she has rated 4 or 5. Presumably, sharing these highly enjoyed activities with others should encourage participants to experience a sense of mutuality and cohesiveness. This approach also provides the opportunity for lively discussion about the different ratings given by members who engage in similar pastimes. As such, this exercise can be a stepping-stone for in-depth discussion about the uniqueness of one's experiences in retirement, etc. Not everyone adjusts the same way, and not every activity is experienced with equal affective meaning.

Leisure ought to be joyful but (unfortunately) for many, it is not. If warranted, people can be asked to compare their lists for areas that show the least enjoyment (ratings 1 and 2). This exercise can open up a discussion of such problem areas as boredom, feelings about adapting to physical limitations, and so on. It can also elucidate areas of unhappiness or dissatisfaction, especially if an individual has many 1 and 2 ratings. The sensitive worker can use this material for an in-depth discussion about areas of psychological apprehension and can encourage problem solving. For example, the group might discuss how individuals can do more of what they enjoy or how they can discover new enjoyments. Sometimes, low ratings involve areas of potential guilt, such as negative feelings about doing things with certain family members. This problem is sometimes better handled in a psychotherapeutic context.

This exercise also lends itself to other structured approaches. Individuals can be asked to sum up the number of activities that they rated 4 or 5 (much enjoyment) and can compare them with the activities that they have rated 1 or 2 (little enjoyment). This procedure can lead to a fuller discussion about how participants feel about their total leisure experiences. Do some rate everything as very enjoyable? How do they manage this? Is it all attitude? Do some have neither much enjoyment nor little enjoyment (ratings of 3)? Do some have mostly little enjoyment? Such an exercise can stimulate helpful support for areas of strength and can lead to problem solving by the group. Many ways of improving or changing one's situation may thus emerge through discussion of the structured material.

The use of enjoyment ratings can also lead to the creation of a *human-resources group*.[16] This group stresses helping members to extend their levels of functioning to the upper limits of their potential. In the human-resources group, the leader focuses on the positive potential that each member has rather than on any pathology. A group leader can use the enjoyment rating scale for such a purpose by focusing discussion on those items that each member most enjoys.

The enjoyment ratings can also be used to help people compare their ideals with the reality of their situations. This can be accomplished by asking participants to review their highly rated enjoyment items and by suggesting that participants indicate how often they actually experienced each particular activity. It has been our experience that people not only put down activities that they have not done for some time (or have done infrequently) but that they also list things that they would like to do but have never done.

The goal of the exercise is to help people to better live up to their ideal self-concept and cope with their real selves. This goal can be approached by using the multiple-strength-perception method or the action-program method.[17]

The *multiple-strength-perception* method essentially requires that one person become the center of the group's attention for a particular session. The "target" person begins by enumerating and sharing with others the strengths that she or he sees in the self as well as the factors in that person's life that might inhibit her or him from using these strengths fully. Other members then discuss their own perceptions with the target person.

The *action-program* method involves having the group encourage a particular member to develop a plan (in addition to talking about what he or she would like to do) that would increase and facilitate the development of the person's strengths. According to Blocher:

> Members then report back to the group the successes or failures in these action programs. When difficulties are encountered, the entire group works to bring their understanding and sensitivity to bear on the problem and so help remove the blocking to further development. Action programs may begin at superficial levels, such as taking art or dancing lessons, and move through to quite significant undertakings, such as developing greater creativity or deeper personal relationships. . . . The use of public commitment and group reinforcement are major sources of gain in this model.[18]

The usefulness of this approach is illustrated by the following: In one group, a participant had listed "playing the piano" as something that she enjoyed greatly. When the worker discussed her various listed activities, it became apparent that the last time that the participant had actually played a piano was some 15 years ago. There was clearly an incongruence between her actual self and her ideal self. When asked why she no longer played the piano, a number of important things emerged. First, it had nothing to do with physical disability. Second, and more important, it had been an activity to which she had given only cursory thought and that she had been timid about revealing her interest to anyone. Yet, it was something that she greatly enjoyed. This exercise permitted her dormant potential to emerge. Once it emerged, group discussion provided the opportunity for others to express interest in her activity. In addition, the participants inquired as to why she had not been playing the piano recently and began to motivate her to develop an "action plan." The other members thus became potential resources. One member recalled that a piano was available in the lounge of the small college where this discussion took place. This led to the group considering how and when the piano could be used by our "target person," not only to play at senior-citizen events, but also to teach others. The group was thus able to activate an interest that had been dormant for some years. It is for this sort of purpose that the enjoyment-rating technique might be most fruitfully used.

Uses for the Activity Gains Form—Assessment of Developmental Experiences Through Leisure. A discussion about what is gained through involvement in various activities listed by participants can lead to reflection about their life experiences in developmental terms. The assessment technique illustrated by the Activity Gains form provides a tangible way of approaching such developmental material. The counselor or worker can use each person's self-assessment to encourage a deeper discussion about life goals. Descriptor phrases can be used to encourage a discussion about developmental life tasks in terms of the subjective experiences of the members. Since the descriptor phrases are worded in terms of positive experiences, they lend themselves for use as part of the multiple-strength-perception and action-program methods.

One important area of life experience that this technique sometimes reveals is the need for intimacy (item 6 on the Activity Gains form). For some, intimacy emerges as a definite strength (in that a number of activities seem to meet this need). For others, it is clearly a significant deficit. We shall focus on this issue for illustrative purposes.

Confiding intimately with someone so that one's personal problems, thoughts, and feelings can be shared is highly important for older people. Kimmel, for example, notes that having a confidant might offset the depressing role loss or decline in social interaction that are often experienced by the aged.[19] The need for intimacy is not necessarily resolved by increased participation in general social-activity programs. As we noted in our discussion about the importance of continuing to have an impact on others, two people can play many games of cards or checkers without necessarily finding out much about each other. This is not to say that social activities for the aged are bad; it is only to say that the functions of these programs are useful but limited.

In light of this, we question why many programs for the elderly seem to focus on implementing the dictates of activity theory. Broadly stated, activity theory involves the idea that "if you keep busy, you stay healthy." This notion, derived from the Puritan work ethic, in conjunction with the wear-and-tear biological theory of aging, suggests that what older people keep busy with is less important than the mere activity of keeping busy.[20] Furthermore, it seems that many older people have internalized this notion. Bengston, for example, quotes a 73-year-old who said that his only life goal was "to keep active—I want to wear out, not rust out."[21] If this attitude is uncritically accepted as typical by workers and programmers for the aged, it may lead to an overemphasis on activity and to a diminished concern with providing relationship experiences that, in the long run, are probably more important for uplifting morale. Lowenthal and Haven, for example, found that older people who maintained a stable intimate relationship evidenced less depression and greater life satisfaction (morale) than did older people who reported having no confidant. Their findings also showed that morale remained high for those older people who had confidants, even if they had suffered decreases in role status or in levels of social interaction.[22]

Intimate relationships provided by a marriage, family, and friends provide satisfaction for people of all ages. Indeed, for persons aged 65 to 74, great emphasis is placed upon satisfactions achieved within marriage and the family.[23] It seems that having someone close gives a person a sense of having an impact upon that person, along with being a significant part of that person's life. This was found in one study, which revealed that, for men, the strongest predictors for life satisfaction in later life were their own characteristics (emotional and physical) and those of their wives. The wife's characteristics were seen as being even more influential on life satisfaction than were their own.[24] It seems clear that the continued experience of having an impact on and with others is very important to the community aged.

We believe that the *confidant*, or *impact, theory,* and its implications, should be more closely followed by those who work with the aged. Broadly stated, this theory holds that keeping busy is important but that being involved in a stable relationship (with someone with whom you can share your activites or feelings about yourself and who will share their feelings with you) is more important. Such needs, and how well they are met, may be elucidated by the developmental-assessment exercise discussed in Phase 4 (see Appendix F).

Uses For the Radius of Activities Form—Ecological Assessment Of Activities. It has often been said that, in old age, one's spatial world shrinks because the environment is not designed to accommodate the needs of older pepole. For example, an older person may have difficulty crossing wide avenues because street lights change too rapidly, while numerous stairs may prevent access to subways or commuter trains. Indeed, research studies show that older people cannot take advantage of many of the numerous facilities available to the younger, more mobile members of the population because the environment is not geared to them.[25] This nonuse of facilities may lead to a spatial shrinking that may be a combined result of socially induced psychological barriers (such as depression related to retirement and caution induced by a nonchallenging environment) and biological deficits associated with aging. Discounts and passes for senior citizens are not always the answer. For example, one person would not use her senior-citizen pass (for public transportation and other available discounts) because the pass symbolized "admitting that she was old." She stopped visiting friends in distant neighborhoods and cut down on going out because she really could not afford to pay the regular transportation fares and other prices on her Social Security income. Some old people may therefore need various forms of remotivational counseling to deal with the more socially induced psychological deficits of spatial mobility.

The information derived from participants who use the Radius of Activities form (see Appendix G) is useful because it provides potential role models for exploring greater parts of the environment. Through discussion with peers, older persons who have confined themselves to a narrow radius might be influenced by members of the group to broaden their activity horizons. Information about what others do can also generate motivation for trying new activities. Discussion of the radius of activities can provide the opportunity for various social learning experiences and can complement the case-centered and human-resources approaches previously discussed. For the young–old, ecological assessment and discussion can serve the function of remotivational counseling. For the more physically impaired, the assessment may help engender reality confrontation and discussion of how to deal with the problems of decreased mobility without giving up one's full exploratory potential. We recall one such discussion in a nursing home that turned into a group planning session on how to arrange for transportation (through administration) for trips to a nearby city, a topic that might not have otherwise emerged.

Public transportation—its difficulty and its high cost—is not always a barrier to exploratory behavior. Carp, for example, concluded that the extensive social isolation found in her study of the elderly in San Antonio, Texas, resulted from the unavailability, as well as the high cost, of transportation in that city. She found that bus service routes were not within easy access and that busses either ran infrequently or did not go directly to the destinations desired by many of the aged in her sample.[26] A study by Bourg in Nashville found a similar situation. He concluded that easy access to transportation was a critical link in the ability of elderly people to remain functional members of society.[27]

Similarly, of 780 New York elderly over 65 years of age who were interviewed, it was found that most of them walked a good deal, both for functional activities (such as shopping) and for leisure activities:

> When asked about what they did each time they left the house during a two-day interval, 56 percent of the trips mentioned were walking trips, particularly for local shopping. Trips that necessitated leaving the neighborhood were infrequently undertaken. Relatives . . . were likely to be visited only once a month, whereas friends, who more often lived nearby, were likely to be visited more frequently. The average person estimated that he could walk about nine blocks to the store without becoming tired.[28]

The foregoing discussion points out that anyone who works with an older population must pay particular attention to the influence of environmental factors on observed behavior. This is especially true if the aim is to help motivate an exploratory attitude. The social learning and role modeling implicit in group approaches may be avenues to achieving such an aim. Short of changing the environment, theme-oriented group discussion approaches (such as the ecological-assessment technique) can help the aged to change dysfunctional attitudes resulting from environmentally and socially induced feelings of decreased competence. In this light, Bengston noted that ". . . an individual's sense of self, his ability to mediate between self and society, and his orientation to competence are related to the kinds of social labeling and valuing he experiences in aging."[29]

Given the sociological fact that the aged are automatically labeled as dysfunctional in our society, we should not be startled to discover that many of our community aged have internalized a sense of incompetence that is evidenced in decreased exploratory potential. Recall, for example, the woman who would not use her senior-citizen pass because it symbolized old age (or incompetence?) which in turn, made her functionally incompetent because she cut down on visiting. In sum, the ecological-assessment technique is one method devised to break this syndrome. It does so by providing the following:

- New reference groups.
- New role models of ecological competence.
- An opportunity for group planning functions in relationship to the environment.

Uses Of the Qualitative Descriptions Of Leisure Experiences. The simplest use of the qualitative description of experiences is that the worker helps develop a sense of communication and understanding among participants about one another's personal lives. The worker or counselor may initiate a group session by suggesting that each participant discuss and share the kinds of things that she or he does with leisure time. It is not necessary to require that each participant refer to his or her list of self-generated activities or evaluation forms. Here, the format can be more freewheeling, in order to encourage general, open discussion. Although this approach is simple, it adheres to the notion of tangible themes because the topic focus can remain on the subject of leisure. The qualitative description approach can be incorporated as part of the discussion of the self-generated-activities list. This is done by suggesting that participants discuss (without referring to any of the forms) and compare what they gain from each of their listed activities.

Phase 8. Individual Counseling and Follow-Up. Although not crucial, it is sometimes fruitful to have ongoing counseling available in order to deal more specifically with issues raised by the leisure discussion exercises and theme groups. We suggest that the worker be prepared to make appropriate referrals whenever the need for more intensive counseling arises. Such referrals should only be suggested, of course, if the participants ask for them. We might also note that, in general, older people (as a group) do not want individual counseling even when it is readily available. In this light, the best modality for follow-up appears to be group counseling or group therapy, or both.[30]

THE PEER-GROUP COUNSELING APPROACH

Another approach to working with the community aged has been developed by Waters, Fink, and White.[31] They note that, over the years, researchers have consistently observed that older people receive a very small share of available psychotherapeutic services. Indeed, it has been suggested that many therapists tend to avoid working with older people because of the anxiety that these clients engender due to their inevitable physical decline. Sargent suggests that therapists tend to be better reassured by working with younger patients.[32] Psychoanalysts, too, have noted the various difficulties that younger therapists have with an elderly population. Grotjahn suggests that younger therapists feel self-conscious or apologetic when they work with clients who are much older than themselves. He suggests that therapists who wish to treat elderly patients must have successfully analyzed their own attitudes toward their own parents and grandparents.[33] Another problem can occur if the therapist becomes unduly idealizing or patronizing with elderly clients. This playing out of the "good" grandchild role may leave both parties uncomfortable. It seems that the best possible attitude for any worker to maintain is one of warm, empathic directness. We believe that anyone who works with the aged should be trained to deal with the potential problem areas discussed above.

In general, it appears that help with maintaining satisfying interpersonal relationships has not been made readily available to the aged, even though many of them report feeling lonely, isolated, and depressed. A group-counseling approach that relies on the use and development of paraprofessional peer counselors has been suggested to meet these interpersonal needs.[34] A peer counselor is someone from one's own age group who is trained to work therapeutically (though often in a limited capacity). A major value of peer counseling is that older counselors often share the same life experiences as their clients. An additional value of this approach is that the peer counselors themselves are often helped in significant ways through the process of being trained to perform a helping function. There seems to be little doubt that, if older community peers are trained to a level of paraprofessional expertise, they can be very helpful in senior-center programs. According to Waters, Fink, and White, "It is difficult for clients to say that they are too old to learn when their group counselors range in age from 55 to 75, and are themselves clearly launched in new directions."[35]

The Continuum Center Model

The peer-group counseling approach originated at the Continuum Center at Oakland University in Michigan. The program has two main purposes: to develop peer-group counselors for the community aged and to provide a direct interpersonal counseling service to the community aged in the Detroit area. The program's principal aim is to help older people deal effectively with issues of loneliness and alienation through the opportunity to share their concerns with others, and to develop new and satisfying relationships through peer interaction.

The Program. The initial phase of the peer-group counseling program is structured. It offers time-limited group counseling in a series of seven two-hour sessions. There are two stages. Following a preorientation meeting, during which the goals of the program are introduced and commitments for participation are made, a series of structured communication skills and values-clarification exercises is presented. For example, group members are asked to place themselves at either of two sides of the meeting room as a way of indicating which of two pairs of words presented by the leader in a series of dyads—such as "Cadillac or Volkswagen," "loner or grouper," "bubbling brook or placid lake"—they are most like. This forced-choice exercise, derived from values clarification, is a technique presumed to motivate self-exploration and to precipitate involvement.[36]

Following these initial exercises, participants are broken up into small, structured groups in which they discuss their reactions to the previous session. According to Waters, Fink, and White:

> [At session two] . . . participants are asked to spend five minutes in the small group talking about people and experiences which have been most significant in their lives, ending with what is most important to them at the present time. This encourages participants to talk about themselves, to focus on strengths they have developed, and to look at and listen to each other. Throughout this exercise, group (peer) leaders model reflective listening.[37]

Subsequent sessions involve similar structured activities that focus on heightening self-esteem and improving interpersonal competence. Participants are encouraged to go on a "*trust walk*," which (theoretically) involves learning how to deal with depending on someone else. The "trust walk" method requires that one member of a pair close his or her eyes while being led by another member of the group. Another typical activity performed by the group is a "*naming*" exercise that requires everyone to state each member's name every time the group meets. This "naming" exercise has been proven to reinforce further learning, for many group members have claimed that they were able to remember all of the names, even though they thought they were too old to learn them. The sessions end with a strength-bombardment activity.[38] In this exercise, each person lists her or his strengths on a piece of paper, and other group members add strengths that they have observed in that person during the program's progress. This technique is another example of a tangible counseling approach to working with the community aged. Unlike the life-enrichment approach, peer-group counseling seems to rely on structured *exercises* instead of structured *themes*.

After having participated in the exercise series, clients are provided with an opportunity for less-structured personal counseling, in order to follow up on any issues raised during the sessions. Waters, Fink, and White report that very few of their elderly clients seek individual counseling but that approximately one-third of them continue in small-group counseling. They suggest that the generally observed reluctance of older people to seek various forms of psychological help may be more related to treatment modality (the form in which treatment is available) than to other factors. Group members are also encouraged to enroll in the paraprofessional training program. Much success is reported with this latter approach.[39] That older persons can be effective paraprofessionals, acting as counselors, was also demonstrated in a recent study whereby older, paid, non-degree-educated persons were trained for one year by a trained consultant, after which they acted as counselors to peers living as community "shut-ins" due to physical disability. The clinical impression reported was that these paraprofessionals, once trained, were most effective in offering their counseling services.[40]

REFERENCE NOTES

1. Neugarten, B., Age groups in American society and the rise of the young old. *Annals of the American academy of political and social sciences*, 1974, *415*, 187–198.
2. Gottesman, L., Quarterman, C., & Cohn, G. Psychosocial treatment of the aged. In C. Eisdorfer & M. Lawton (Eds.). *The psychology of adult development and aging*. Washington, D.C.: American Psychological Association, 1973.

3. Herr, J. J., & Weakland, J. H., *Counseling elders and their families*. New York, Springer Publishing Co., 1979, pp. 64–68.
4. Brok, A. J. Existential instrumental and developmental issues in leisure relevant to counseling and applied human development. *Society and Leisure*, 1976, *3*, 61–71.
5. Waters, E., Fink, S., & White, B. *Peer group counseling for older people*. Paper presented at the 83rd annual convention of the American Psychological Association, Chicago, Ill., 1975.
6. Palmore, E., George, L., & Fillenbaum, G. Predictors of retirement. *Journal of Gerontology*, 1982, *37*, 733–742.
7. Guntrip, H., *Schizoid phenomena, object-relations and the self.* New York: International Universities Press, 1969.
8. Lilly, J. C. Mental effects of reduction of ordinary levels of physical stimuli on intact, healthy persons, In H. M. Proshansky, W. H. Ittelson, & L. G. Rivlin (Eds.), *Environmental psychology: Man and his physical setting,* 1st ed. New York: Holt, Rinehart, & Winston, 1970.
9. Gottesman, Quarterman, & Cohn, Psychosocial treatment of the aged.
10. Maddi, S. R. The search for meaning. In W. J. Arnold & M. M. Page (Eds.), *Nebraska symposium on motivation*. Lincoln: University of Nebraska Press, 1970.
11. Brok, A. J., Free time and internal-external locus of control: Is socialization for freedom dignified?'' *Society and Leisure*, 1974, *6*, 121–128.
12. Brok, A. J. Existential instrumental and developmental issues in leisure relevant to counseling and applied human development.
13. Wallach, M., & Kogan, N. *Modes of thinking in young children*. New York: Holt, Rinehart & Winston, 1965.
14. Erikson, E. H. *Childhood and society*, 2nd ed. New York: W.W. Norton & Company, 1963.
15. Starr, B., & Weiner, M. B. *The Starr-Weiner report on sex and sexuality in the mature years*. New York: McGraw-Hill, 1982.
16. Blocher, D. H. *Developmental counseling*, 2nd ed. New York: The Ronald Press, 1974.
17. Ibid.
18. Ibid., pp. 219–220.
19. Kimmel, D. *Adulthood and aging*. New York: Wiley, 1974.
20. Kuypers, J. A., & Bengston, V. L. Social breakdown and competence. *Human development*, 1973, *16*, 181–201.
21. Bengston, V. L., *The social psychology of aging*. New York: Bobbs-Merrill Company, 1973, p. 6.
22. Lowenthal, M. F., & Haven, C. Interaction and adaptation: Intimacy as a critical variable. *American sociological review* 1968, *33*, 20–30.
23. Cutler, N. E. Age variations in the dimensionality of life satisfaction. *Journal of gerontology*, 1979, *34*, 573–578.
24. Mussen, P., Honzik, M. P. & Eichorn, H. Early adult antecedents of life satisfaction at age 70. *Journal of gerontology*, 1961, *16*, 134–143.
25. Lawton, M. P., & Nahemow, L. Ecology and the aging process. In Eisdorfer & Lawton (Eds.), *The psychology of adult development and aging*.
26. Carp, F. Public transit and retired people. In E. J. Cantilli & J. L. Schnelzer (Eds.), *Transportation and aging: Selected issues*. Washington, D.C.: Administration of Aging, 1971.
27. Bourg, C. *Life styles and mobility patterns in older persons*. Paper presented at the Interdisciplinary Workshop on Transportation and the Aging, Administration on Aging, Washington, D.C., May, 1970.

28. Lawton & Nahemow, *Ecology and the aging process*, p. 656.
29. Bengston, *The social psychology of aging*, p. 47.
30. Waters, Fink, & White, *Peer group counseling for older people*.
31. Ibid.
32. Sargent, S. S. Therapy and self-actualization in the later years via nontraditional approaches. *Psychotherapy: Theory, research and practice*, Winter 1972, *19*(4), 522–531.
33. Grotjahn, M. Analytic psychotherapy with the elderly. *Psychoanalytic review*, 1955, *42*, 419–427.
34. Waters, Fink, & White, *Peer group counseling for older people*.
35. Ibid., p. 10.
36. Simon, S. B., Howe, L. W., & Kushenbaum, H. *Values clarification*. New York: Hart Publishing Co., 1972.
37. Waters, Fink, & White, *Peer group counseling for older people*, p. 6.
38. McHolland, J. *Human potential seminars*. Evanston, Ill.: Kendall College, 1972.
39. Waters, Fink, & White, *Peer group counseling for older people*.
40. Weiner, M. B., & Pamilla, T. M. *Case management training of older community workers: Implications for extended outreach*. Paper presented at the XIII International Congress of Gerontology, New York Hilton, New York, July 12–17, 1985. (Abstract: *Book of Abstracts*, XIII International Congress of Gerontology, p. 307.)

13

General Issues in Psychotherapy for Older People

In previous sections, we have discussed several group approaches, such as the modalities of "the stepladder approach." These techniques were originally designed to include only those elderly living within an institutional setting and considered "frail." We have also discussed some approaches for the community elderly.

In this section, we discuss the process of psychotherapy as a special, distinct technique. For the most part, this type of approach is geared to the "active" elderly—the person who is living in the community, is relatively independent, is mentally active, and has the motivation or desire to uncover, explore, and understand some life-long conflicts or, as the case may be, some relatively new or situation-related conflicts. It is thought that it is the motivation for change, within both the therapist and the client, that is the predictor for "cure," and not age itself that is crucial to the psychotherapy process.[1]

Since psychotherapy is intense and involves high-level cognitive ability, along with the paying of fees (whether modest or high), it is usually considered a "higher-order" form of treatment and is geared essentially to the active elderly. The approach that we will outline is the traditional, or psychoanalytically-oriented, one. Unlike supportive therapy (described earlier in Chapter 10), in which the goal is the promotion of a more satisfying life without any attempt at personality reorganization, this approach necessitates an understanding (on the therapist's part) of defense mechanisms and focuses primarily on the major underlying processes of transference and resistance. Again, unlike supportive approaches, in which defenses and life-long conflicts are not tampered with, a goal of traditional therapy is to understand defenses and to deal with them. The eventual aim is to "change defenses" as a way of altering personality and, in this way, provide the client with a happier, more satisfying existence.

We will describe both individual and group treatment approaches, with the understanding that *only* trained persons, whatever their orientation, are equipped to practice psychotherapy. Once such training has been achieved, the rewards of working closely in therapy with an older adult can be most exciting. We now explore some pertinent issues.

ASSETS OF AGE

Since Freud, clinicians have discussed the difficulties of employing successful psychotherapeutic treatment with older people. Even so, there are many qualities that emerge in later life that actually support the therapeutic process. Older people have often achieved a comfortable status in life and are less concerned with *what they do* than with *who they are* as people.[2] Later life, for some, provides ample time for introspection and for consideration of inner experience. These are both important conditions for successful psychotherapeutic treatment.

It has also been noted that certain character traits may be more easily treated in later life. People who are overly self-preoccupied, as in pathological narcissism, who are unable to be concerned with others, and who seem incapable of responding empathically or are unduly exhibitionistic may be more amenable to treatment in later life.[3] The demands of reality, which younger people may more easily deny, may finally be accepted by the older person. It is as if the sands of time are slowly grinding down the rock-like, rigid personality structure. Later life sometimes softens and opens those previously unmoved by life experience.

The acceptance of shortcomings related to aging is an important life task. A pathological inability to do this is noted by Kernberg:

> A woman in her middle fifties who dressed and acted as if she were a late adolescent became aware during treatment of how afraid she was that younger women would deprecate her for being old and spent, as she had deprecated older women when she was young and beautiful. But she was even more concerned at losing the sense of triumph over her contemporaries.
>
> She had the illusion that she was still the youngest among them and the most attractive—and if she dressed appropriately for her age, other women would triumphantly enjoy the breakdown of her superiority. She could not go back to visit her home town, her family and friends of the distant past, because they all would notice how much she had aged, while they, living together, would be oblivious to their own aging.[4]

In contrast, Kernberg[5] describes the normal, nonpathological way of dealing with the shortcomings of aging. This, he notes, is characterized by the ability to maintain autonomous interests while accepting dependence and external support under conditions of stress or when objectively needed. In particular, the ability to maintain an emotional investment in areas that are no longer under one's control is a crucial consequence of normal—in contrast to pathological—narcissism. Says Kernberg, "The aging person who can still love being in the mountains when he can no longer climb them illustrates this point."[6]

For those in psychotherapy, a life-long struggle with reality may help soften entrenched character defenses. The environment, in effect, becomes the therapist's silent partner. In sum, the aged client brings many strengths and assets to the therapeutic experience. Given the client's maturity, he or she is often able to take a thoughtful, objective view of the self and of others while accepting human frailties and vanities.

TREATMENT TECHNIQUES

In general, psychotherapy with older people requires some modification of traditional technique. This is due, in part, to the fact that the older adult, raised in a different era, shares certain common characteristics. For example, the older person is generally less educated in, and not as familiar with, psychological jargon as are younger persons. A therapist working with the older person should be aware of this and should choose terms that are understandable. For example, rather than using abstractions or generalizations, one must be prepared to be more concrete. The authors have found, in their own practices, that what proves useful is giving examples or anecdotes with which the client can relate, particularly as they apply to the client's own life experience.

As with all clients, one begins treatment by asking the person to talk about her- or himself. This allows the therapist to formulate an idea of what the client is all about, to reach some tentative diagnostic understanding (is it mainly depression, is it a narcissistic disturbance?), and to gain some clues as to how the interaction (transference) between client and therapist is most likely to take place. The history that the client shares with the therapist provides the background for how to work and where to focus.

Kahana[7] suggests that the treatment focus should be on a *current* problem that the client consciously recognizes. He also stresses that the client should be given a readily perceivable part in solving his or her own problems.[8] This latter approach is in keeping with the *action-program* method discussed earlier in this volume.[9] The only difference here is the importance of understanding the transference development for the sake of appropriate therapeutic management.

Dealing with Transference

Transference is a unique type of relationship with a person. "The main characteristic is the experience of feelings to a person which do not befit that person and which actually apply to another. Essentially a person in the present is reacted to as though he were a person in the past . . . It is an anachronism, an error in time." It also involves a displacement: "impulses, feelings, and defenses pertaining to a person in the past have been shifted onto a person in the present. It is primarily an unconscious phenomenon, and the person reacting with transference feelings is, in the main, unaware of the distortion."[10]

In addition to the above, older people may be prone to a special kind of transference when they are working with a younger therapist. They may distort the relationship so that the therapist is experienced as a son or daughter and may relate to the therapist in a paternalistic or maternalistic manner. We feel that real age differences must be respected to be able to maintain a successful working relationship but that the therapist who is treated as a child by a "parent–client" needs to be aware that this may be a defensive maneuver to allay anxiety about feeling dependent on the therapist.[11]

Transference reactions may be positive or negative. They are never neutral! A client may have warm thoughts about the therapist and may consider him or her the most wonderful person in the world, knowledgable, and perfect. Though a portion of these feelings may be based on reality, they also reflect what might be called an idealized-positive transference. The therapist is seen as all-knowing, as incapable of any wrong or error. Aspects of a positive transference are important to maintain a good working relationship with the client, and some newer approaches encourage full acceptance of the idealization.[12] When these feelings are extreme, however, traditional approaches maintain that they are defensive and will ultimately lead to great disappointment in the treatment, if neglected.

Negative transference is precisely the opposite. Such clients mistrust the therapist, feel angry toward him or her, and maintain a noncooperative stance in the treatment. Indeed, in extreme cases, negative transference often causes a client to leave treatment prematurely, without understanding the distorted nature of her or his reactions. To a moderate degree, some negative transference is welcome in therapy. It means that the person is capable of accepting flaws in the therapist and is willing to accept his or her own negative and positive feelings toward people.

Clients experiencing negative therapeutic reactions, which may occur after the therapist "speaks hopefully to them or expresses satisfaction with the progress of the treatment, . . . shows signs of discontent, and their condition invariably becomes worse."[13] In effect, such people appear to get worse during the therapy treatment instead of getting better. This reaction is often related to the client's need to sustain a transference tie with the therapist. Often, patients repeat past negative experiences. Some recreate in their present lives relationships similar to those with important others in their past. The therapist may find him- or herself cast in the role of a parent that previously and consistently failed to support the client.

The sensitive therapist can help work through the negative response by being aware that she or he (the therapist) may have indeed failed the client in a given situation, by not being sufficiently empathic or by having failed to tune into the client's needs and feelings at a critical moment in the client's experience. The client needs to feel that his or her subjective experience is confirmed and validated by the consistent empathic understanding of the therapist.[14]

Many psychotherapists who work with older people say that it is preferable to emphasize the positive aspects of the therapeutic relationship while minimizing negative feelings. Kahana[15] suggests that, although difficult material should not be deliberately avoided, the therapist clearly should make "no attempt to rekindle old conflicts." This means that "the therapist is active in providing guidance, reassurance, and environmental manipulation . . . (and) educational techniques may be used."

Similarities to Treatment of Narcissistic Clients

A striking similarity exists between treatment recommendations for the older person and the narcissistic person. The importance of the working relationship and of empathy, and the use of active techniques in a supportive environment, are to be stressed in therapeutic work with both types.

PROBLEMS FACED BY THE CLINICIAN

> Although I had been engaged in clinical work for almost 25 years, the kinds of problems these people asked about were not the kinds of problems to which I was accustomed. One difference was that very often they were not problems that could be resolved or eliminated. Rather, they were problems to which the person had to learn to adapt.[16]

These words express what the average clinician often observes when face-to-face with an older client or group. What are some of the problems and concerns presented by older people?

Increasing Loss of Autonomy

An older man felt depressed because he realized that he ought not to drive at night because of his failing night vision. Yet, this was the only way that he could get to the center of town to visit his grandchildren and to eat dinner with his busy son and daughter-in-law. Since they came home from work late, they could not readily drive the 22 miles to his house to pick him up and return to their apartment. Eighty-two and active, he preferred to live in a small village on the outskirts of the larger town where he had lived for the past 50 years. He could tend his vegetable garden and enjoy doing other physical work. The amicable relationship that he enjoyed with his son and daughter-in-law had been based on his ability to drive to their apartment without needing help. Now, he faced the experience of being unable to visit them except on special occasions, when they could drive out to pick him up. His other choice was to move into a nursing home closer to town, but it seemed silly to him, since he was in good health except for his night vision. Though he could still drive in the daytime, this was also becoming an issue. Even though he could arrive at their apartment in the daytime, he would still need to be driven home at night, a 44-mile round trip. The couple clearly could not make this long a trip on a regular, three or four times weekly, basis.

Children

The foregoing example also highlights issues that older people face in relation to their children. Older people are often stressed by the problems of their children. If not redefined, the role of being a parent may engender severe emotional difficulties. One astute clinician notes that "the older parent may be just as emotionally troubled over the problems of their adult children as over the difficulties of young and dependent children. With the young child, the parent may take action, while with the adult child, the parent is usually at a loss as to what to do beyond offering emotional support.''[17]

Loss of Important Personal Relations

Although new relationships can be formed in later life, it is perhaps a developmental task to accept that one cannot replace the experience of being with someone who ''knew you when you were young and with whom you shared many significant memories.''[18] Older persons are sometimes fearful of new experiences. ''Everyone seems to have their network of friends, and I don't know how to break in to form new friendships'' is a typical expression of the older person's dilemma.

GROUP THERAPY

Group therapy is a dynamic mode of psychotherapeutic treatment to employ with older people. In some ways, the group approach is an ideal one as regards dealing with issues faced by the elderly (such as the need for forming new relationships). A stimulating group experience addresses both the need to continue feeling a sense of significance in relation to others and the importance of challenge in daily life. Further, a good group offers opportunities for modeling and for understanding how others cope with problems similar to one's own. The sense of acceptance, renewal, and warmth offered by an active, working group process can be of incomparable value to the older person.

A sensitive treatment group allows the sharing of one's accumulated wisdom with others. At the same time, one's defensive habits are examined, observed, and clarified. Through this approach, one's sense of self is encouraged and is prodded to grow, even as one's personal limitations are accepted by the group.

History

Group therapy for the elderly initially emerged as a technique used primarily for geriatric patients. As a treatment of choice, the use of groups was first viewed as a way of treating large, diverse populations not otherwise accessible through individual psychotherapy. The application of the group modality to elderly institutionalized patients focused on the necessity of treating growing numbers of older adults with organic or functional disorders.[19] Supportive, leader-centered groups emphasizing the development of daily living skills were considered more important than groups focusing on the development of insight and personality change.[20]

With an increasingly older population, the American public and health professionals are increasingly aware of the needs of the healthy elderly. Recent trends include the development of group psychotherapy and other group-treatment methods for those elderly who are not living in institutions. Programs for the healthy elderly, such as the SAGE project, skills training (for example, assertiveness training), and the peer–helper concept, have proven very useful.[21-23] In general, flexible theme-oriented support groups, such as leisure counseling, widowhood, and reminiscence groups, have been considered most effective.[24-26]

The Psychotherapy Group

Although all groups may be therapeutic, the psychotherapy group is marked by an intensive psychodynamic approach. While such a group may include supportive therapies and skill development, the psychodynamic therapy group emphasizes interpersonal relating, insight, and personality development. The phenomena focused upon in these groups are the same for all age groups. As previously stated regarding individual psychotherapy, issues that arise in the group must be related to the particular needs of the aged. We call this the *same–difference* problem.[27] Older people are the same . . . but are also different . . . from younger people. The clinician must therefore always be aware that working with older patients calls for supporting them in their efforts to adapt to current life conditions and to meet the challenges of their changing lives. As in individual treatment, the psychotherapy group deals with both change and adaptive functions.

Why "Group"?

What makes group therapy such an important therapeutic modality? What is it about the group dynamic that makes it an effective treatment-of-choice? This section will compare both group and individual treatment methods.

Existential Issues. In individual treatment, patients understand that they will be listened to exclusively by the therapist. No other person will interrupt or challenge their right to the therapist's full attention. In group therapy, however, this exclusive right is not guaranteed. Each group member must establish his or her *presence*, carve out an identity within the group, make her- or himself known—assert, even, that his or her self exists! From the very first encounter, group members must decide whether their thoughts or comments are relevant or significant enough to warrant the group's attention. The group sets up priorities together, and an agenda is developed. It is as if each patient thinks, "Am I important enough to interrupt the discussion of the other patients, or should I wait? Can I contribute? Should I start the group? Am I significant enough to be listened to?" The act of choosing to establish one's position in relation to others is an important therapeutic event; indeed, it is the very fabric of the group dynamic. For the older person, the process of establishing oneself as a significant member of the group may either stimulate stressful feelings or lead to an exhilarating feeling of independence. The discovery that one's ideas and feelings may have priority and often have significance and meaning to others enhances self-esteem and nurtures feelings of worth.

Development of Empathy. More than any other therapeutic modality, group therapy helps one to develop a keener sense of empathy. By empathy, we mean the capacity to feel joy for another's happiness and sadness for another's distress. In general, empathy requires that a person be able to clearly understand, and identify with, others. To empathize is to put oneself "in another person's shoes," to actually feel what they are feeling. This is a basic cornerstone for mature interpersonal relations.

Let us compare the difference between individual and group treatment in terms of the person's need to be empathic. In individual treatment, it is unlikely that the therapist will someday tell the client, "I feel great today. My wife bought me a wonderful present," or "Let me tell you about the new house I'm building." It is also unlikely that the therapist would tell her or his client, "Look, I feel depressed. Can you listen to what happened to me today?" Appropriately, most therapists are carefully trained to be warm and authentic with their patients but not to use the client's time for their own needs or gratification.

In group therapy, however, the above exchanges are regular occurrences. The therapist's task is to help group members improve their ability to appreciate, and react genuinely to, each other's experiences. The opportunity for reciprocity and sharing between members in a group is lacking in the structure of the individual-treatment relationship.

For a preoccupied or self-involved older patient, sharing may be a difficult task. In the group dynamic, others' appreciation for one's empathy with them provides meaning and validation for growing intimacy, even strengthening one's connection with others. Through empathy, the group also provides the opportunity to realize that one can still offer nurturing and companionship to others in an appreciated way.

Corrective Emotional Experience. Being a group member provides the chance to experience direct feedback, admiration, and pleasant observations. Members learn self-worth from comments such as "You look so good today" or from direct, positive feelings like "I really enjoy being with you." A special response might be, "I appreciated what you told me in the previous session. It helped me a lot." These comments toward a client would normally be more restrained by a therapist in an individual session.

Some Typical Problems Suitable for Group Therapy

Seventy-one-year-old Tess retired some six years ago from a life-long civil-service job. She had never married and had devoted her attention to work. Upon her retirement, she pursued a bachelor's degree in art history at a local university that gave her advanced standing for "life experience." (Such a pattern for physically healthy older adults has become more prevalent in urban areas throughout the country in the past decade.) Having pursued this interest in art to develop her "aesthetic side," Tess now feels depressed. Just graduated, she still does not have close friends, even though she lives in an urban setting and is active and physically healthy. An acquaintance suggests that Tess see a therapist at a local community clinic. At the clinic, the suggestion is made that group treatment might help Tess learn to interact more and understand why she fails to make friends despite the fact that people initially find her interesting. Tess is motivated because she does not wish to feel isolated and because she realizes that group treatment may help her to develop long-inhibited social interests.

Jack, a 68-year-old engineer, lost his wife to cancer six months ago. His two grown children live in faraway cities and have their own families. Jack has the choice of living with either one of his children but does not particularly wish to give up his work, as he is not required to retire until he is 75. He has been feeling depressed, however, and has been drinking excessively at night. His physician refers Jack to a psychiatrist for antidepressant medication. The psychiatrist decides that Jack could do well in interactive group psychotherapy, particularly if the group has some members who have gone through a bereavement period. It is hoped that Jack can share his pent-up feelings and can learn from others who have dealt with similar losses.

Lazlo, 75, emigrated from Hungary after the 1956 revolution and developed his own construction business with his two sons. One of his sons died in Vietnam. The remaining son now feels that he should run the business, since his father suffered a stroke two years ago. Lazlo gets into bitter disputes with his son and compares him negatively with his deceased brother. Lazlo's wife constantly worries that he will succumb to another stroke and also pressures him to retire. As a result, Lazlo moves out of his house and into a motel. He feels isolated and lonely but continues to live in the motel for a full year while still running his business. Eventually, he moves back home, retires, and feels "ill at ease." Although his health remains stable, he becomes progressively more withdrawn, despite his wife's desire to travel with him and despite her social resources and friendships. He becomes irascible with his wife and talks of living in a motel again. The physician at his HMO recommends group psychotherapy, asserting that his health is as good as may be expected, given his medical history.

Treatment Benefits of Group Therapy

How can these older people, and others, benefit from a psychotherapy group? Yalom outlined some of the curative factors of the process and makes the following observations about work with the aged:[28]

Instillation of Hope. One of the advantages of belonging to a therapy group is the exposure to fellow "travelers" who are on the road to improvement. The presence of other people who are coping effectively with problems similar to one's own can inspire, uplift, and rekindle hope. This process may be evoked through identification and sets the stage for new behavior. The term *identification* suggests the "taking in" of another's experience for the sake of one's own learning and growth. Many group therapists have had the experience of hearing clients remark at the end of treatment how important it was for them to have observed the improvement of others. Yalom notes:

> Group therapists should by no means be above exploiting this factor by periodically calling attention to the improvement that members have made. Therapy group members themselves proffer spontaneous testimonials when new, unconvinced members enter the group.[29]

The older patient, in particular, may respond well to being with peers who have learned to cope with illness, the loss of a spouse, new goals after retirement, and other problems.

A word of caution: The composition of the group is important in situations where crises are dealt with. As social–psychological research shows, situations that arouse fear or provoke too much anxiety can lead to defensive denial and can inhibit progress.[30] A relatively healthy older person recuperating from a minor operation ought not to be included in a group composed of patients suffering from more serious impairments or from life-threatening illnesses.

Universality. Many people feel as if their problems are unique and live in what can be termed "pluralistic ignorance."[31] Their very isolation may heighten their feelings of being the only one facing a difficult situation. Yalom writes:

> . . . because of interpersonal difficulties, opportunity for frank and candid consensual validation in an intimate relationship are [*sic*] often not available to (these) patients. In the therapy group, especially in the early stages, the disconfirmation of their feelings of uniqueness is a powerful source of relief.[32]

In perceiving their similarity to others, and by sharing their deepest concerns, patients often benefit from the resulting catharsis and, ultimately, from acceptance by other members of the group.[33] For the elderly, this can be a powerful healing influence. For example, the discovery that one's difficulties with one's children are not at all unusual may relieve anxiety or feelings of failure that are intensified by the belief that one is the only parent who "does not feel appreciated." In sharing the universal nature of parenthood, experiencing both its problems and its triumphs, a group member may find relief in sharing burdens and failures, as well.

Frequently, older people have difficulty letting go of their now-mature children and accepting their children's personal autonomy.

In a recent group, 60-year-old Sam, who recently became a grandfather, had been having differences with his daughter-in-law. She felt that he was too intrusive with his advice about how she and her husband should raise their new son. Sam's own son supported his wife in this argument and, as a result, the grandfather felt unappreciated. In the group, Sam reported the following dreams, illustrating his conflict and his efforts to resolve them through regressive wishes that he projected onto his son.

> I was cleaning wax with a Q-tip from my ear because I could not hear well. I began to feel I couldn't do it and began calling for my son. He appeared and did it for me, and I felt great.

Sam's conflict dealt with listening and communicating with others (the wax in his ears), precisely his difficulty in group! In a similar way, he had difficulty "listening" to his children. Sam's passive wish, as expressed in his dream, makes his position obvious! He would listen—and clean the wax from his ears—only if his son did the work for him!

In the group, those members with feelings similar to Sam's could identify, and deal, with their roles as adult parents. Others expressed the wish to remain in charge (not be separated from their children), as well as the longing for someone to take care of them.

Imparting Information. Information-giving is a vital, curative part of group therapy. It is usually experienced indirectly, except in a highly-structured group, where didactic information is part of the process. In addition to providing useful information, didactic instruction can lower anxiety.

Advice-giving, in and of itself, is not very useful in a psychodynamically oriented therapy group. When it occurs with regularity, it indicates that the group is either very new or is in a state of resistance and has regressed to an earlier mode of interacting. A member who gives advice with regularity, to the exclusion of sharing his or her feelings and experiences, is possibly avoiding the therapeutic task. In giving advice, some find a false sense of security, by abandoning the given role of working group member and adopting the position of auxiliary therapist.

Yalom notes that "the process of advice-giving, rather than the content of the advice, may be beneficial, since it implies and conveys a mutual interest and caring."[34] This is the positive aspect of advice-giving, and it may lead to a greater sense of significance and self-worth. As a pattern, however, we feel that it is too often used as a defense against sharing one's personal feelings.

The therapist who primarily imparts information, rather than prodding members to share feelings, may inadvertently be encouraging group resistance and defensiveness. The more structured and leader-centered the group is, the more likely it is that patients will imitate this behavior. This can lead to a "super-ego" group atmosphere, each patient identifying with the role of therapist rather than with fellow group members.

Altruism. Participation in a group encourages the development of empathy, promoting shared experience in far greater measure than the typical diadic exchange between client and therapist. Similarly, the group dynamic enhances and nurtures altruistic feelings toward others. Feelings of worth, the experience of one's own power and significance—of having made an impact on another—can heighten self-esteem and can heal habits of low self-evaluation.

A client hearing the gratitude of others in the group may experience her- or himself in new and meaningful ways. When one client tells another, "I'm glad of what you told me last week. I thought about it, and I think you're right," the experience may be enlightening and strengthening. Such learning experiences are particularly relevant to the isolated elderly, many of whom have lost loved ones toward whom they could express their altruistic and nurturing feelings. Group therapy offers growth opportunities through giving, enhancing feelings of significance central to an inner sense of well-being.

Encouraging the Development of Personal Control. The psychotherapy group is structured to encourage its members to solve their own problems through reflection and a better understanding of oneself. Rather than a process of giving advice, a working group dynamic promotes a spirit of shared inquiry. Research suggests that older people who are more active feel more in control of their circumstances and are more successful in coping with their problems. These elderly are less likely to feel depressed.[35] As one 80-year-old group member put it, having a sense of being "in charge of our life," of being able to come to terms with one's life and its conditions—a coming of age, wherever one may live—is an accomplishment well worth achieving at any age.

REFERENCE NOTES

1. Weiner, M. B., & Wilensky, H. A psychotherapeutic approach to emotional problems of the elderly. *Journal of Nursing Care*, May 1978, 14–18.
2. Wheelwright, J. B. Some comments on the aging process. *Psychiatry*, 1959, *22*, 407–411.
3. Kernberg, O. F. *Internal world and external reality*. New York: Jason Aronson, 1980, p. 149.
4. Ibid, p. 141.
5. Ibid.
6. Ibid.
7. Kahana, R. J. Strategies of dynamic psychotherapy with the wide range of older individuals. *Journal of Geriatric Psychiatry*, 1979, *12*, 71–101.
8. Ibid.
9. Weiner, M. B., Brok, A. J., & Snadowsky, A. *Working with the aged*. Englewood Cliffs, N.J.: Prentice-Hall, 1978, pp. 187–188.
10. Greenson, R. R. *The technique and practice of psychoanalysis*. New York: International Universities Press, 1967, pp. 151–152.
11. Goldberg, A. *Negative therapeutic reaction in the future of psychoanalysis*. New York: International Universities Press, 1983, p. 335.
12. Kohut, H. *How does analysis cure?* Chicago: University of Chicago Press, 1984.
13. Ibid.
14. Ibid.
15. Kahana, R. J. Strategies of dynamic psychotherapy with the wide range of older individuals, p. 74.
16. Swensen, C. H. A respectable old age. *American Psychologist*, March 1983, *38*(3), 328.
17. Ibid., p. 333.
18. Ibid.
19. Parham, I. A., Priddy, J. M., McGovern, T. V. J., & Richman, C. M. Group psychotherapy with the elderly: Problems and prospects. *Psychotherapy: Therapy, Research, and Practice*, Winter 1982, *19*(4), 437–443.
20. Ibid.
21. Lieberman, M. A., & Gourash, N. Evaluating the effects of change on the elderly. *International Journal of Group Psychotherapy*, 1974, *29*, 283–304.
22. Corby, N. Assertion-training with aged populations. *The Counseling Psychologist*, 1975, *5*, 69–73.
23. Waters, E., White, B., Oates, B., et al. *A peer group counseling for older people*. Rochester, Mich.: Oakland University Continuum Center, 1979.
24. Weiner, M., Brok, A., & Snadowsky, A. *Working with the aged*, Chapter 4.

25. Hainer, J. Groups for widowed and lonely older persons. In B. MacLennan, S. Saul, & M. B. Weiner (Eds.), *Group therapy in the mental health treatment of the elderly*. New York: International Universities Press. (In press.)
26. Lewis, M. I., & Butler, R. N. Life review therapy: Putting memories to work, in individual and group psychotherapy. *Geriatrics*, 1974, *29*, 165–173.
27. Brok, A. J. Some thoughts on the education of youngsters about aging and the aged. *Proceedings of the 4th Annual Conference on Life-Long Learning*. New York State Association of Gerontological Educators, October 12, 1976, New York, N.Y., pp. 61–68.
28. Yalom, I. *The theory and practice of group psychotherapy* 2nd ed. New York: Basic Books, 1975.
29. Ibid., pp. 6–7.
30. Janis, I. L., & Feshbach, S. Effects of fear-arousing communications. *Journal of Abnormal and Social Psychology*, 1953, *48*, 78–92.
31. Moscovici, S., & Zavalloni, M. The group as a polarizer of attitudes. *Journal of Personality and Social Psychology*, 1969, *12*, 125–135.
32. Yalom, I. *The theory and practice of group psychotherapy* 2nd ed.
33. Ibid., p. 9.
34. Ibid., p. 2.
35. Kahn, R. L., & Antonucci, T. C. Applying social psychology to the aging process: Four examples. In J. Santos & E. R. VandenBos (Eds.), *Psychology and the older adult: Challenges for training*. Washington D.C.: American Psychological Association, 1982; Michaelson, R. R., Michaelson, C. B., & Swensen, C. M., *Factors related to coping strategies employed by older adults*. Paper presented at the meeting of the American Psychological Association, Washington, D. C., August, 1982; Swensen, C. H. A respectable old age, *American Psychologist*, 1983, *38*(3), 328–334.

14

Teaching the Community About the Aged

ALTERNATIVES TO INSTITUTIONALIZATION

The vast majority of elderly people live in the community, yet they are stereotyped as senile people who are institutionalized. More often than not, these stereotypes are reinforced in the media. In addition, stories about "good" care in a facility seldom make news, but scandals are ensured a place on page one. Much of the current focus in the field of aging is on providing alternatives to institutional care. As stated earlier, only a very small proportion of the elderly are institutionalized. For the majority of the elderly, therefore, the home and the neighborhood are the central locations in their lives and are the appropriate foci for the provision of services.

Traditionally, the elderly have been expected to bring themselves to whatever service programs are offered, but they have not always come. There are many reasons for this: pride; lack of knowledge; expensive and inconvenient public transportation; bureaucratic barriers, such as eligibility requirements for services; long waits at clinics and at other agencies; insensitive attitudes on the part of those who render services; fragmentation of services; and, most important, gaps in the current service-delivery system. To date, therefore, many well-intentioned, well-funded programs have been woefully underutilized.

It should be stressed again that all aging people, although chronologically similar, are distinct individuals who have varied and unusual skills, abilities, and problems. Interventions must, therefore, be based on understanding this distinctiveness. It is apparent that there is a need for a whole spectrum of services that would allow for individual adaptations by providing a range of options. One of the primary advantages of living in the community is that one has access to more options than does someone who lives within the closed system of a residential-care facility. A major goal, then, would be to maintain this independence by providing the aging in the community with support services that would allow them to function optimally.

An advantage to this approach (one that is very seldom recognized) is that the cost of maintaining the aging person in the community is generally far smaller than is the cost of providing the total services of an institution. Since health-care budgets are limited, more services could be dispersed among more people in the community, thus stretching health-care dollars. Moreover, this approach places the focus of services in the home and neighborhood, precisely where the target population is located.

Pathology in the Community

It is generally recognized that less than 2 percent of the community elderly use mental-health services of any kind. Recent emphasis has been on emotional behaviors related to organic brain syndrome; this is sometimes called senile dementia and is identified as the disease that most closely resembles the stereotype of old age. As stated elsewhere, this usually refers to cognitive dysfunction characterized by loss of short-term memory and by impaired judgment and disorientation. It has been found that one-half of all senile dementia is due to Alzheimer's disease, the remainder being caused by multi-infarct (stroke), Pick's disease, and other types of diseases.[1] While there is much research being conducted on "senile dementia/ Alzheimer's type" (SDAT), there is still much that we do not know. What has been determined is that this is a major psychiatric disturbance of old age, characterized by a "deterioration of higher-order cortical functions," which underlie the "symptom complex which characterizes this type of dementia."[2]

While reported rates of "senile dementia" vary, some recent statistics suggest an overall estimate of 6.6 to 9 percent for those 65 and over; prevalence rates for moderate to severe dementia in the community (noninstitutionalized) are between 4 and 7 percent. There are basic differences between age groups, however. For those over 75, the estimates for affliction are less than 5 percent, but for those over 80, the estimates more than double (12 percent). With the onset of dementia, each of those afflicted may respond differently to the illness, largely depending upon personality and response modes throughout life. Behavioral symptoms of dementia include suspiciousness, paranoia, acute anxiety, panic, passivity, agitation, and hostility.[3] In diagnosing senility, Terry L. Brink says that physicians have a responsibility "to explain in greater detail to the concerned children of aging patients that there are more than four dozen organic disorders which can produce a confusional state in later life, and that modern means of assessment, although imperfect, are adequate in most cases." He points out that the time taken to explain the basis of a medical diagnosis does much to strengthen the credibility of medical staff and to improve relations with client families.[4]

In the past few years, there has been increasing recognition that the aged experience the same mental and emotional disorders as do younger persons, though probably more frequently. It is hypothesized that the increased incidence of mental and emotional problems may be related to the increasing number of stresses and losses that are experienced with increased age. Many mental-health difficulties of the elderly are largely treatable, however, as they are in younger groups. As with any community group, the worker must be sensitive to the presence of such symptoms as depression, anxiety, and addiction. In addition, the worker must be sensitive to the myriad stresses that can precipitate emotional crises, such as financial problems, physical problems, bereavement, forced retirement, malnutrition, and isolation. Very often, symptoms can be correlated with these external stresses and can be alleviated with appropriate interventions, such as medical treatment, drugs, counseling, and psychotherapy. Before treatment can be offered for emotional problems, however, there must be a thorough physical and psychosocial assessment by qualified professionals. It must be emphasized once again that each older person is an individual. The worker should thus be alert to the fact that *aging itself is not a disease* and that many of the problems of aging are treatable. Recognition of problems, and referral to appropriate personnel, are important services that the worker can provide.

NEEDS OF THE ELDERLY

In this century, we have seen a tremendous increase in life expectancy and, therefore, a dramatic increase in the number of elderly in our society. We have not, however, seen a concomitant increase in our concern for the well-being of this segment of the population. In fact, at least 25 percent of those over 65 are now living below the poverty level, and many more are hovering around it, constantly struggling to make ends meet.[5]

Related to this is the fact that we are a youth-oriented society and, as such, we try to deny aging as much as possible. The elderly who manage to look and "think" young fit in. The others remain invisible and often isolated, with both groups tending to perpetuate our society's denial of aging. Nowhere is this more apparent than in the realm of public policy. Simply put, when it comes to aging, we have none! And there has yet to be a coordinated effort to change this. Programs and services remain fragmented and inadequate. For example, Social Security legislation was designed to meet the post-Depression crisis of the 1930s, not to be the primary source of postretirement income that it is today. Medicare insurance was intended to make more, and better, health care accessible to the elderly regardless of income but, in reality, it now covers less than one-half of the annual out-of-pocket health expenditures of today's elderly and has fallen far short of its goal.[6] A multitude of similar examples can be drawn from many existing programs and services.

What, then, is needed? A sound public policy must be devised that would establish a government commitment toward making changes to improve the lot of the elderly. Their needs would determine what programs and services would be established and offered. Basically, there is a need to establish a total range of options that would ensure aging people the support necessary for them to maintain themselves in the community and to have, as much as possible, a continuity of lifestyle.

Comprehensive Services

A network of comprehensive services would include simultaneous medical, social service, personal service, and environmental interventions. Available options would form a spectrum of services based on needs ranging from minimal interventions, such as one-time information and referral ("I and R") services, to institutional placement for total care. In devising this network, the following should be considered:

1. Because of the realities of increasing physical and mental frailty with increasing age and the fact that many elderly are (at some point) on a downhill course, there must be recognition of a *long-term need for services*. The kind of service may have to be altered as conditions change. But, no matter what the service, the goal would ensure optimal functioning, however limited this might appear. The services would range from simple preventive care, such as routine health screenings, to the total care of the skilled nursing facility (SNF).
2. Realistic *goals must be set*. In working with the elderly, goals are often relatively limited. For example, a young stroke victim may be rehabilitated to engage in contact sports, but a frail elderly person may only be rehabilitated to walk again with the help of a walker.
3. *Options must be provided* to account for individual differences. For example, housing alternatives might include single-family dwellings, apartment living, hotels, assisted apartment living (services offered in the building), communes, the British type of supervised housing (called "warden housing"), or other forms of congregate living, the most extreme being the nursing home or mental hospital. Simple activity opportunities might include the range of commercially available recreation opportunities; organizations (such as church groups or clubs of retired people); public programs (such as senior-citizen centers); day care programs; or volunteer work and employment programs.
4. There is a need for *outreach*. A fact to be considered is that many elderly remain invisible and therefore isolated. These people are often the target population for services, but they are rarely reached. The elderly do not generally seek out services; therefore, services must be brought to the elderly. Those who provide services must be mobile and must be able to bring the services to neighborhoods and even to the home. An example might be a mobile crisis intervention team. For example, a team of mental-health professionals, which might include a psychiatrist, nurse(s), social worker(s), and other professionals and paraprofessionals, could go to the home of a distraught, emotionally troubled aging person who will not leave the house despite the efforts of caring family, friends, and neighbors.
5. There is a need to *link services*, and someone must take the initiative in coordinating them. Currently, fragmentation is a tremendous problem. For

example, an elderly client who has both physical and emotional difficulties may be treated simultaneously by several doctors who have no communication with, or even knowledge of, one another. A possible consequence is that the client may be placed on contraindicated medications. In addition, since no one physician is involved in total care, and since the client may have no family and no significant others, the need for homemaking services is overlooked in the shuffle. As a result, the client may feel psychologically fragmented, and thus, further stress may be added. In this case, a social worker, nurse, or paraprofessional staff person at a community agency may serve as a liaison, and expensive duplication of services can be avoided. This samc pcrson could also provide advocacy services for the elderly client unable to fend for her- or himself.

THE ELDERLY PERSON AS A SELF-ADVOCATE

Most elderly people would be their own advocates if given the opportunity. The complexities of the current services system and the limited education and limited mobility of many of our elderly make self-advocacy extremely difficult. This is compounded by the fact that so many of today's aging persons were raised in an era in which activism was frowned upon as being "rabble rousing," so they passively accept their lot. (This is in contradistinction to the dynamic activists who champion the rights of the elderly and are known as the "Gray Panthers.") In addition, there is a tendency for many professionals and laypersons to treat the elderly as nonpeople or, at best, to infantilize them—to treat them as though they were children (note the common stereotype of the old person regressing to "second childhood"). Instead of listening to the client and acceding to his or her wishes, decisions and services are inflicted upon the client. Consequently, many elderly are forced into being dependent. The more the dependence is encouraged, the more dependent they become, thus creating a vicious cycle.

To break this cycle, a massive program of education about aging is indicated. Such a program should include a generalized education, which would start with young children and would present aging as a developmental stage not very different from other stages in the life cycle. Special efforts should be made to reach middle-aged persons and to encourage them to actively attempt to improve the lot of their parents while simultaneously assuring a better future for themselves. Again, professionals and paraprofessionals currently working with the aged could, and should, serve as change agents in this process. Most of all, the elderly themselves should be included in this process, because they can help dispel some of the negative stereotypes and myths about aging by providing direct evidence of the positive attributes of aging, which can be maximized through *direct interaction* between the aging person and the community at large. To educate for *aging* is to educate for *life*.

REFERENCE NOTES

1. Weiner, M. B., Teresi, J., & Streich, C. *Old people are a burden but not my parents.* Englewood Cliffs, N.J.: Prentice-Hall, 1983.
2. Emery, O. B., & Emery, P. E. *The dementing process in senile dementia Alzheimer's type.* Paper presented at the XIII International Congress of Gerontology, New York Hilton Hotel, New York, July 12–17, 1985.
3. Weiner, Teresi, & Streich. *Old people are a burden but not my parents.*
4. Brink, T. L. The myth of the "senility myth." *Journal of the National Medical Association*, 1980, *72*(11), 1042.
5. Brotman, H. B. Who are the aging? In E. W. Busse & E. Pfeiffer (Eds.), *Mental illness in later life.*
6. Butler, R. *Why survive?* New York: Harper and Row, 1975.

Appendices

Evaluation Forms

A

Geriatric Rating Scale

Instructions
Rate each patient by circling a zero, one, or two after each item. The *higher* the score, the *less* intact is the patient's functioning. Thus, a high score (many ratings of 2) would indicate that a patient is functioning poorly and could be assigned to a rehabilitative program, such as sensory training. Where the patient's scores fall in the medium range (many ratings of *1*), he or she might be assigned to a program such as reality orientation. A total score that includes many zeros might indicate an approach such as remotivation or activity therapy.

Patient's Name ______________________________
Rater's Name ______________________________
Date ______________________________

Circle *only* the number that applies

1. When eating, the patient requires:			
No assistance (feeds self)	0		
A little assistance (needs encouragement)		1	
Considerable assistance (spoon feeding, etc.)			2
2. The patient is incontinent:			
Never	0		
Sometimes (once or twice per week)		1	
Often (three times per week or more)			2
3. When bathing or dressing, the patient needs:			
No assistance	0		
Some assistance		1	
Maximum assistance			2

	Circle *only* the number that applies		
4. The patient will fall from his bed or chair unless protected by side rails:			
Never	0		
Sometimes		1	
Often			2
5. With regard to walking, the patient:			
Has no difficulty	0		
Needs assistance in walking		1	
Does not walk			2
6. The patient's vision, with or without glasses, is:			
Apparently normal	0		
Somewhat impaired		1	
Extremely poor			2
7. The patient's hearing is:			
Apparently normal	0		
Somewhat impaired		1	
Extremely poor			2
8. With regard to sleep, the patient:			
Sleeps most of the night	0		
Is sometimes awake		1	
Is often awake			2
9. During the day, the patient sleeps:			
Sometimes	0		
Often		1	
Most of the day			2
10. With regard to restless behavior at night, the patient is:			
Seldom restless	0		
Sometimes restless		1	
Often restless			2
11. The patient's behavior is worse at night than in the daytime:			
Never	0		
Sometimes		1	
Often			2

	Circle *only* the number that applies		
12. When not helped by other people, the patient's appearance is:			
Almost never sloppy	0		
Sometimes sloppy		1	
Almost always sloppy			2
13. The patient masturbates or exposes her- or himself publicly:			
Never	0		
Sometimes		1	
Often			2
14. The patient is confused (unable to find way around the ward, loses possessions, etc.)			
Almost never	0		
Sometimes		1	
Often			2
15. The patient knows the names of:			
More than one member of the staff	0		
Only one member of the staff		1	
None of the staff			2
16. The patient communicates in any manner (by speaking, writing, or gesturing) well enough to be easily understood:			
Almost always	0		
Sometimes		1	
Almost never			2
17. The patient reacts to his or her own name:			
Almost always	0		
Sometimes		1	
Almost never			2
18. The patient plays games, has hobbies, etc.:			
Often	0		
Sometimes		1	
Almost never			2

	Circle *only* the number that applies		
19. The patient reads books or magazines on the ward:			
Often	0		
Sometimes		1	
Almost never			2
20. The patient will begin conversations with others:			
Often	0		
Sometimes		1	
Almost never			2
21. The patient is willing to do things asked of him:			
Often	0		
Sometimes		1	
Never			2
22. The patient helps with chores on the ward:			
Often	0		
Sometimes		1	
Never			2
23. Without being asked, the patient physically helps other patients:			
Often	0		
Sometimes		1	
Almost never			2
24. With regard to friends on the ward, the patient:			
Has several friends	0		
Has just one friend		1	
Has no friends			2
25. The patient talks with other people on the ward:			
Often	0		
Sometimes		1	
Almost never			2
26. The patient has a regular work assignment:			
Away from the ward	0		
On the ward		1	
No regular assignment			2

	Circle *only* the number that applies		
27. The patient is destructive of materials around her or him (breaks furniture, tears up magazines, etc.)			
Never	0		
Sometimes		1	
Often			2
28. The patient disturbs other patients or staff by shouting or yelling:			
Never	0		
Sometimes		1	
Often			2
29. The patient steals from other patients or staff members:			
Never	0		
Sometimes		1	
Often			2
30. The patient *verbally* threatens to harm other patients or staff:			
Never	0		
Sometimes		1	
Often			2
31. The patient *physically* tries to harm other patients or staff:			
Never	0		
Sometimes		1	
Often			2
Total score ( )			

B

Sensory Training Evaluation

The following is a modified outline of the sensory training evaluation form. It was compiled with an interdisciplinary team at the David Minkin Rehabilitation Institute, Brooklyn, New York.

Instructions

At the end of *each* session, please rate the patient on each of the areas listed. The highest number (2) indicates the best level of response and the lowest (0) the poorest level of response.

Patient's Name ______________________ Age ____ Sex ____

Leader's Name ______________________ Ward ________

Job Title ____________________ Date ____ Session No. ____

Does the patient speak English? well ____ poorly ____ not at all ____

	(2) Usually	(1) Sometimes	(0) Never
1. Identification of body parts (can identify by touching or verbalizing)	________	________	________
2. Recognition of different odors (recognizes by saying: "this is sweet," "bitter," etc.)	________	________	________

	(2) Usually	(1) Sometimes	(0) Never
3. Awareness of different textures (can identify a piece of rough cloth, a piece of velvet, etc.)	______	______	______
4. Auditory acuteness (attentive when others are talking)	______	______	______
5. Visual attentiveness (looks at leader or other members when appropriate)	______	______	______
6. General interest in others (appears interested in leader or in others)	______	______	______
7. General interest in environment (notices things around him or her)	______	______	______
8. General enjoyment (seems to enjoy being with others)	______	______	______
9. General participation (shows attempts to participate in group)	______	______	______
10. General positive adaptation (e.g., is not disruptive in group)	______	______	______
		Total score* (	)

*To get the total score, give a weight of (2) to a rating of ''usually'' and a weight of (1) to ''sometimes'' and add all the scores.

The leader of the group should keep track of changes in these scores over time as a way of denoting progress or decline (see next page). In addition, test scores may indicate early deterioration and a need for additional supportive measures.

Check Statement that Applies
Since the last report, has patient shown any

(a) improvement in meetings? Yes ____ No ____
(b) improvement on the unit? Yes ____ No ____

Final Report for Series
Initial score (first session) ____________________ Date ____________
Final score (sixth session) ____________________ Date ____________

Check off the following:
____ Promote to higher-level group (e.g., Reality Orientation)
____ Continue in the same group for another six-session series
____ Transfer to another group
____ Inactive (to be reassigned)

Note: At final session of series, place this form on patient's chart.

C

Reality Orientation Evaluation

The following is a modified outline of the Reality Orientation Evaluation Form. It was compiled with an interdisciplinary team at the David Minkin Rehabilitation Institute, Brooklyn, New York.

Instructions

At the end of *each* session, please rate the patient in every area listed. The highest number (2) indicates the best level of response and the lowest (0) the poorest level of response.

Patient's Name ______________________ Age_____ Sex_____

Leader's Name ______________________ Ward__________

Job Title ______________________ Date_____ Session No._____

Does the patient speak English? well_____ poorly_____ not at all_____

---

	(2) Usually	(1) Sometimes	(0) Never
1. Orientation to person (knows who he or she is)	________	________	________
2. Orientation to place (knows where he or she is)	________	________	________

	(2) Usually	(1) Sometimes	(0) Never
3. Orientation to time/date/day (knows the time of day, names the day, etc.)	______	______	______
4. Verbal communication (responds to or initiates verbal exchange with others)	______	______	______
5. Social behavior (recognizes group leader, smiles in recognition, extends hand, nods, etc.)	______	______	______
6. General interest in others (appears interested in leader or in others)	______	______	______
7. General interest in environment (notices things around him or her)	______	______	______
8. General enjoyment (seems to enjoy being with others)	______	______	______
9. General positive adaptation (e.g., is not disruptive in the group)	______	______	______
10. General participation (shows attempts to participate in group)	______	______	______
			Total score* ( )

*To get the total score, give a weight of (2) to a rating of "usually" and a weight of (1) to "sometimes" and add all the scores.

Changes in scores over time denote progress or decline. In addition, early deterioration may be noted and additional intervention measures introduced.

Check Statement that Applies
Since the last report, has patient shown any

(a) improvement in meetings? Yes ____ No ____
(b) improvement on the unit? Yes ____ No ____

Final Report for Series
Initial score (first session) ______________________ Date ____________
Final score (sixth session) ______________________ Date ____________

Check off the following:
____ Promote to higher-level group (e.g., remotivation)
____ Continue in the same group for another six-session series
____ Transfer to another group
____ Inactive (to be reassigned)

Note: At final session of series, place this form on patient's chart.

D

Remotivation Evaluation

The following is a modified outline of the Remotivation Evaluation Form. It was compiled with staff members of an interdisciplinary team at the David Minkin Rehabilitation Institute, Brooklyn, New York.

Instructions
At the end of *each* session, please rate the patient on every area listed. The highest number (2) indicates the best level of response and the lowest (0) the poorest level of response. Do this *as soon after* each session as possible.

Patient's Name ____________________ Age_____ Sex_____

Session No. ____________________ Ward No.______ Date______

Remotivator ____________________ Topic________

Job Title ____________________

---

	(2) Usually	(1) Sometimes	(0) Never
1. Interest	______	______	______
2. Awareness	______	______	______
3. Participation	______	______	______
4. Comprehension	______	______	______
5. General enjoyment	______	______	______

Total score* (   )

---

*To get the total score, give a weight of (2) to a rating of ''usually'' and a weight of (1) to ''sometimes'' and add all the scores.

Check Statement that Applies

Since the last report, has patient shown any

(a) improvement in meetings?	Yes ____	No ____
(b) improvement on the unit?	Yes ____	No ____

Final Report for Series

Initial score ______________________________ Date ______________

Final score (sixth session) ______________________________ Date ______________

E

Self-Generation of Leisure Activities

Age ____________

Sex ____________

Instructions

List below the kinds of things that you do in your leisure time. Put down anything that comes to your mind. The order in which you write these activities is not important. After you have listed everything that you can think of, rate each activity according to a scale of enjoyment, from *1* to *5*, where *1* is the low end of the scale and *5* is the high end of the scale. Circle the number that best expresses your degree of enjoyment.

Leisure Activities	Place	Degree of Enjoyment Little				Much	Gains
A		1	2	3	4	5	
B		1	2	3	4	5	
C		1	2	3	4	5	
D		1	2	3	4	5	
E		1	2	3	4	5	
F		1	2	3	4	5	
G		1	2	3	4	5	
H		1	2	3	4	5	

Leisure Activities	Place	Degree of Enjoyment Little				Much	Gains
I		1	2	3	4	5	
J		1	2	3	4	5	
K		1	2	3	4	5	
L		1	2	3	4	5	
M		1	2	3	4	5	
N		1	2	3	4	5	
O		1	2	3	4	5	
P		1	2	3	4	5	
Q		1	2	3	4	5	
R		1	2	3	4	5	
S		1	2	3	4	5	
T		1	2	3	4	5	

F

Activity Gains

1. This activity gives me the feeling that other people support me in my interests. My confidence in others is affirmed.
2. This activity gives me freedom to be separate and a sense of standing on my own two feet. This activity reinforces my belief of being able to take care of myself.
3. This activity gives me a chance to explore and to be creative. I enjoy this activity because there are no set rules. I decide what the activity consists of and how I will do it.
4. This activity gives me a sense of accomplishment and helps me to gain a sense of achievement.
5. This activity helps me to learn more about myself and to find out who I am. It gives me a chance to try different ways in which to do things and by which to discover new things about myself.
6. This activity allows another person to find out more about me and encourages me to find out more about another person in depth. It involves sharing meaningful feelings with another. Through this activity, I get close to another person and expose my personal side.
7. This activity allows me to feel that I am contributing something worthwhile to others or to society. This activity helps me to feel that I am giving something, helping others, or making my mark on another person's life, on an organization, or on a community.
8. Through this activity, I can appreciate the differences between people and can accept myself and others. This activity helps me to feel satisfied with the manner in which I have led my life.

Check off the following:

_____ Promote to higher-level group (e.g., discussion)
_____ Continue in the same group for another six-session series
_____ Transfer to another group
_____ Inactive (to be reassigned)

Note: At final session of series, place this form on patient's chart.

G

Ecology Format—Radius of Activities

Instructions

On the first page, you have provided me with a number of activities that you do in your free time. Please note next to the activity the locale (place) in which you would normally do this activity. Choose from the list of eight places below. You may use a place as often as you like or not at all.

1. Home
2. On my block
3. Within a five-block area of home
4. Neighborhood
5. Other neighborhood in town or city
6. State
7. Outside the state
8. Outside the United States

Index